Homoe

Tomás Pablo Paschero
MD

Edited for publication
by Patricia Haas, MD

Translated from *Homeopatía*
by Katherine V. Masís, MA

BEACONSFIELD PUBLISHERS LTD
Beaconsfield, Bucks, UK

Email: books@beaconsfield-publishers.co.uk
Website: www.beaconsfield-publishers.co.uk

Original edition published by Editorial 'El Ateneo', Buenos Aires, Argentina 1983
This edition © Beaconsfield Publishers Ltd 2000
Translation © Katherine Masís 2000

British Library Cataloguing in Publication Data
Paschero, Tomás Pablo
 Homoeopathy. – (Beaconsfield homoeopathic library; no. 21)
 1. Homeopathy
 I. Title II. Haas, Patricia
 615.5'32
 ISBN 0–906584–41–8

The Publishers would like to express their thanks and appreciation to Katherine Masís, MA for her scholarly translation of this complex book; to Rosalind Shapiro, RSHom for detailed prepublication editorial work; and to Jemima Kallas, LCH for preparing the general index.

Phototypeset by Gem Graphics, Trenance, Cornwall
in 10 on 12pt Times.
Printed and bound in Great Britain by Halstan & Co. Ltd, Amersham.

Foreword

This first English edition of Dr Tomás Pablo Paschero's *Homeopatía* fulfils a wish long cherished by those he trained at the Escuela Médica Homeopática Argentina throughout his life as a homoeopathic physician. Today his chosen students are entrusted with the responsibility of continuing to spread his teachings throughout the small and yet at the same time wide world of homoeopathy.

This book encompasses the whole of his working life. As he says in his Preface, one notices 'the course of a formative process which entailed the development of a Hahnemannian concept of chronic disease ...' And it is precisely that process which was the source of two clear-cut stages in his life – those of a teacher and the director of a school.

The first stage ran from 1933, when he founded the Asociación Médica Homeopática Argentina, along with those colleagues whom he cites and with whom he forged great friendships, until 1969. During those thirty-six years he developed all that is most valuable and profound in his doctrine, as well as his rare ability to interpret homoeopathic remedies as constitutional types. But in 1969 he realised that a group of teachers in his school disagreed with him, sometimes openly, regarding his criteria of teaching. Faithful to his principles and encouraged by a greater number of teachers and students in his school, he decided in 1972 to establish the Escuela Médica Homeopática Argentina, which today carries his name.

Far from being negative, the results of this schism have been beneficial: both of the schools founded by him are on friendly terms, and even though they subscribe to different teaching criteria, they are at one in their efforts to spread homoeopathy.

In his last sixteen years, without obstacles of any kind, Paschero worked as a teacher and contributed enormously to the training of more teachers at his Escuela Médica, allowing them the freedom to research, create and teach, and during this period over fifty physicians graduated from the three-year programme of the school. His students, now experienced teachers, continue to spread his knowledge through books, journals and courses taught throughout Europe and the Americas.

Since then, Dr Paschero's school has consolidated the knowledge contained in his book *Homeopatía*. His lectures, case histories and weekly seminars with us allowed us to analyse and expand on the essence of his thought from many different perspectives.

Because of all this, these selected chapters on clinical practice, doctrine and materia medica are the essence of Paschero's work, a genuine legacy indeed for all those who are proud to be part of his school.

Dr Eugenio Federico Candegabe
Honorary President
Escuela Médica Homeopática Argentina Dr Tomás Pablo Paschero

Preface

This book gathers together a selection of the writings published during the course of a personal formative process which entailed the development of a Hahnemannian concept of chronic disease, and which led to an understanding of homoeopathic remedies as constitutional types. These writings also reflect the influence that the process had on the unfolding of my vocation.

Any profession, no matter how humble, offers the possibility of satisfying a quest for the meaning of life, as long as it is practised with integrity. Thus the dignity of the task depends on who carries it out and how it is carried out, rather than what is actually done. Precisely because humility is required, the art of medicine is an occupation of the highest spiritual order. Medicine consists not only in following the professional rules of the art, but also in transcending them to develop that sense of community which confers a true human sense to one's mission.

This requirement motivated my first steps in medicine. Pondering the meaning of my role vis-à-vis my patients, I began to inquire into the nature and meaning of the diseases from which they suffered. It was not long before I felt that something basic was missing from a training which enabled me to diagnose the pathological lesion, the organic dysfunction or the localised disease. And yet, however exhaustive the symptomatic analysis, it yielded no enlightened synthesis of the whole patient – the very protagonist of their own existential drama whose anguish and moral suffering took the form of subjective symptoms that had no assigned clinical value. I felt ashamed of my inability to respond to the complaints of patients who – intuitively aware of the relationship between their symptoms and their disease – were hinting at a medicine of which I was ignorant and asking for help I could not give.

Again and again I remembered the words of Claude Bernard (1813–78), the great master of experimental medicine, when he said, 'All live phenomena are, beyond doubt, explainable mechanically, but not the order which joins them.' Scientifically oriented medicine lacks a vision of the aetiology of the morbid process in the patient's emotional disturbance, what Hippocrates and those of the Aesculapian School so often extolled – the holistic understanding of the patient – which caused them to say that there are no diseases but only diseased people.

Drawn to this clinical vision and favoured by a chance circumstance, I made my first contact with homoeopathy through Samuel Hahnemann's *Organon*. I felt that this was to be my path on reading the first paragraph, which states: 'The physician's high and *only* mission is to restore the sick to health, to cure, as it is termed'. And further, the third paragraph:

> If the physician clearly perceives what is to be cured in diseases, that is to say, in every individual case of disease ... if he clearly perceives what is curative in medicines, ... and if he knows how to adapt, according to clearly defined principles, what is curative in medicines to what he has discovered to be undoubtedly morbid in the patient ... as also in respect to the exact mode of preparation and quantity of it required (*proper dose*), and the proper period for repeating the dose; ... *then he understands how to treat judiciously and rationally, and he is a true practitioner of the healing art.*

A reflective reading of Hahnemann's *Organon*, Kent's *Lectures on Homoeopathic Philosophy* and Phatak's work helped me to define my spiritual and professional approach. I then had the good fortune to meet Dr Enrique Bonicel, a French pharmacist with a deep knowledge of homoeopathy who had established a homoeopathic pharmacy in Buenos Aires. He generously informed me on the bibliography and preparation of remedies, and also sought out and gathered together the few physicians who, in an isolated fashion, had begun to practise homoeopathy in Argentina: Drs Godofredo Jonas, Jorge Masi Elizalde, Carlos Fisch and Armando Grosso, the latter being an intern at the Children's Hospital. Before long, Drs Grosso, Fisch, Masi Elizalde and I had established a friendship held fast by our yearning to deepen our knowledge and be worthy of the dignity of a homoeopath.

This book summarises what I learned from these three dear and wise friends, now gone but still vibrantly present as teachers and physicians. The same applies to Drs Jonas and Rodolfo Semich, also members of this group of homoeopaths that offered its first lessons at the lecture hall of the newspaper *La Prensa*, to a rapidly growing audience of physicians. Encouraged by our success we established the Asociación

Médica Homeopática Argentina, whose legal status was conferred almost immediately.

During this period I also corresponded with foreign doctors, especially from the United States of America, where Kent, Allen, Farrington, Hering and the other great masters of homoeopathy had written the materia medicas with which I was now familiar.

I then decided to visit the Flower Homeopathic Hospital in New York where I stayed for a couple of weeks, keeping in close contact with such renowned homoeopaths as Drs Stearns, Mackenzie, Elizabeth Wright Hubbard, Jackson and others. I then went to the Hahnemann College of Philadelphia where I was able to practise homoeopathy in a hospital setting, mainly with Dr William Griggs, the renowned homoeopathic paediatrician, who shared his valuable teachings with me. I worked too in Philadelphia with Dr Underhill, who also gave me generously of his time and affection.

At the end of my stay in Philadelphia, Dr E. Dixon, the director of the hospital and with whom I had had lunch daily, gave me an enormous quantity of books which were later to become part of the library of the Asociación Médica Homeopática Argentina. These books are a true bibliographic treasure, as many of them have long been out of print. After a visit to Boston I then travelled to Washington, where I attended many scientific meetings of which I have fond memories and where I had the privilege of working for several days in the private office of Dr Julia Green, one of Kent's students. Finally, I went to Chicago in search of Dr A. H. Grimmer, who had been chief clinician and consultant to Kent himself and who was the main reason for my trip to the United States.

Dr Grimmer welcomed me with a stern yet inquisitive frown. After fixing his gaze on me and hearing my appeal, he curtly explained that he first had to assess my readiness and personal qualities for the practice of homoeopathy. In his long career, he said, he had seen many physicians who had turned out to be bad homoeopaths, due both to a lack of qualifications and honesty, thus harming a system which required steadfast moral and intellectual values as well as a true sense of vocation. Enthusiastic about fulfilling this requirement to the best of my ability, I underwent a thorough examination on homoeopathic doctrine – and I also asked, as a corollary of a prolonged interrogation which he admitted satisfied him, to be allowed to examine a patient and draw up a clinical history before him.

The outcome was that Dr Grimmer invited me to his home, thirty miles from Chicago, and from that moment I worked by his side for four months in his office. I lunched with him daily, and after our work we would retire to his home where his wife and children treated me as a member of the family. After dinner we would retire to his desk, where we would discuss the case histories of the day. I enjoyed his wise explanations which, in his warm and fatherly tone, fulfilled my yearning for knowledge and enriched me spiritually.

I am indebted to Dr Grimmer, a worthy and profound teacher who honoured me with his friendship. To this day I treasure the memory of his strength and integrity. I can still see him standing in the snow on the platform of the lonely railway station, slowly waving his hand, on the night I took the train away. With tears in my eyes I saw him grow more and more distant until he was lost for ever in the shadow of the night. The memory of people like Dr Grimmer, who lived in the service of others, endures in our hearts.

Grimmer has not died, just as Hahnemann, Kent, Hering, Allen, Clarke, Boenninghausen, Roberts, Nash and many other brilliant teachers have not died. They have handed down that humanistic homoeopathy with a spiritual meaning which was present in their own lives. Only by realising the highest values is it possible to practise a medicine such as Hahnemannian homoeopathy, which requires a grasp of the essential symptoms of the patient as a whole, unique and singular human being. These values can be perceived and described only when the physician has discovered his or her own true self.

This is the formative process of the first period of my homoeopathic career which I mentioned at the beginning of this preface and which runs through these writings implicitly, both in those on doctrine and in the materia medica.

I am indebted to my friend Dr Shuji Murata, a distinguished homoeo- pathic physician of our school, for collecting the clinical case histories in this book with zeal and intelligence. I also wish to express my gratitude to Drs Alfonso Masi Elizalde and Eugenio F. Candegabe, special and firm friends, true representatives of Hahnemannian homoeopathy in Argentina, who have encouraged and accompanied me in my teaching endeavours.

T.P.P.

Contents

Chapter 1

Fundamental Principles
(1955)

Armed with the authority that clinical knowledge brings, every homoeopathic physician must take up the mission of defending the value of Hahnemann's principles. But in order to be able to do so, he or she must be aware of two main points – the assimilation of homoeopathic principles and a certain level of self-awareness.

In relation to the first point, the homoeopath must fully understand why the principle *Similia similibus curentur* is the corollary of the Hippocratic aphorism *Natura morborum medicatrix*.

Disease is a process of adaptation to the environment, to the social and biological world that surrounds the individual. This adaptation is not only instinctive but is also produced by intelligence – the ability to decide, reason, and assess circumstances – which is why disease, or adaptation, is a problem of freedom.

It is no longer possible to think of the problem of disease as a localised phenomenon. Life can exist only as a totality, and this totality is based on an imponderable factor which can only be called 'the psyche'. Personality is grounded in the psyche and it is there that the homoeopath must seek the elements necessary for diagnosis. Modern clinical practice needs to consider each patient as a distinct, unique individual case and try to discover their personal traits, without pigeonholing them within pathology or a certain generic type. It is in the study of the psyche – that is, the personality which represents the whole individual – that homoeopathy finds its particular therapeutic role.

Hahnemann does not begin his *Organon* by expounding the law of similarity for the application of homoeopathic remedies, but by pointing out that the one and only lofty mission of the physician is to cure. He maintains that in order to cure a patient, the physician must understand the biological and emotional maladjustment within that individual's environment as a process involving the whole person.

Analytic medicine has developed to the fullest the system of differential diagnosis. However, it is not capable of synthesis, nor of the

1

holistic and unifying clinical perspective necessary for understanding each individual patient. How is it possible to study the human being as an abstraction, as a segregated organism, in complete isolation, with no sense of a biological and emotional relationship with the world? Homoeopathy constructs no theoretical speculation about the condition or disease process from which the patient suffers. Instead, it makes a therapeutic diagnosis based on the personal traits of the individual and the way he copes with life.

Homoeopathy's fundamental premise that disease is a reaction of the whole organism is clearly Hippocratic. There are two diametrically opposed concepts to explain what we call 'disease'. Hippocrates (?460–?377 B.C.) established that disease (*nosos* in Greek) is a way that a person falls ill. On the other hand, the English physician Sydenham (1624–89) thought of disease as a morbid phenomenon of nature that was imposed on the individual. Hippocrates' concept is essentially anthropological: disease is a reaction, which calls for inquiry into the individual mode of response of each patient. Universalising and generalising his observations, Sydenham's approach is clearly scientific and considers the nature of bodily diseases.

The law of cure is a necessary corollary of the holistic principle which guides homoeopathy. It traces the path of vital energy from the centre to the periphery, from the mind to the organs, from vital organs to less vital organs, from the upper part of the body to the lower part, and fulfils itself in the individual's progression towards full maturity – the aspiration of every human being. Only those who adhere to the law of cure in every case that they treat may rightly call themselves homoeopaths.

Psychologically, we reach maturity as human beings when we transcend the self-centred phase – where we try to manipulate people and events according to our own self-interest – into an altruistic, objective stage in which we acknowledge the reality and needs of others as much as our own, realising that we are not single units separated from the rest of life. In homoeopathy, the patient is considered as a whole person who, as his personality evolves, develops adaptive responses to his environment.

These principles form the doctrinal basis of the homoeopath's clinical education, but the homoeopath must also have a certain amount of self-awareness. Physicians who do not perceive or who do not want to face their own subconscious motivations may well create difficulties in their work. They must be mature human beings, able to understand, love and empathise with their patients' problems. Such encounters between physicians and their patients are essential, for it is in this way that physicians gain both an intimate knowledge of their patients' lives as well as a better understanding of their own personal lives.

The physician must be able to empathise with the patient to stimulate their intuition, which will be made up of their own experience of the self, the memory of the symptom pictures they have studied, and the synthetic clinical perspectives that remain as representations in their unconscious mind.

Only thus, by comparing the physician's own life of the psyche with what happens in the intimacy of the patient's psyche, will it be possible to provide a comprehensive clinical practice based on an authentic desire to cure. We do not desire what we previously considered of value – we value that which we desire. Therefore, the principle that leads to the better understanding of each physician's own vocation is absolutely essential.

Chapter 2

Clinical Experience and Remedy Selection
(1943)

The most important moment in clinical practice is when the homoeo-path sees the patient for the second time and thereupon decides on a future course of action. Assessing the data provided by the patient, the physician not only corroborates the diagnosis and prescription but is also in a position to consider the prognosis quite accurately. But in order to do so, he or she must be familiar with certain philosophical concepts to be able to identify what is significant.

To know whether and how effectively a remedy is working is not as easy as it seems. The homoeopath's perspective differs from the ordinary perspective in that the evidence for therapeutic action rests completely on the patient's unique subjectivity, expressed in various ways. The soundness of the data will be proportional to the sharpness of the prescriber's reason and perception.

It is important that the homoeopath has a clear understanding of the principles that Hahnemann and his disciples formulated in assess-ing the morbid process. If the ultimate goal is the patient's cure, we must adhere strictly to established procedures. Thus the homoeopath becomes the direct agent of the law of cure if he practises with integrity and confidence.

When a remedy has been prescribed correctly, the patient may present at the follow-up with few or no objective changes, albeit with clear signs of subjective changes. The patient feels better in himself but the physical symptoms may persist, although slightly ameliorated. Similarly, the patient's mental symptoms may also persist, although to a lesser degree, and the objective signs may remain the same. On the whole, the patient reports feeling better, emotionally stronger and has faith in the treatment. Such a patient would have chronic disease and a complex clinical history and will have resorted to homoeopathy after many years of conventional medical treatment.

If the physician works according to the homoeopathic law of cure, he knows that symptoms must not be treated or suppressed but that the patient's whole symptom picture must be taken into account, creating a hierarchy from the mental symptoms to the particular. Likewise, the homoeopath knows that it is essential to understand the patient's essential dynamic process and, finally, that the therapeutic reaction which follows the law of cure's centrifugal path must be accepted as authentic – that is, from the mind to the organic periphery.

In this way the homoeopath directs and gauges the patient's dynamics and perceives the changes which have been produced. Organic or symptomatic medicine works only on the phenomenal plane. It is here that we see the result of illness, which is really a dynamic disturbance. Homoeopathy, instead, works from within the causal plane of life.

The homoeopath then must always wait for what Hahnemann and thousands of observers subsequently have pointed out – the disappearance of symptoms in the reverse order of their appearance. Hering confirmed and added to this law, stating that under the influence of the homoeopathic simillimum, symptoms disappear following a path from centre to periphery, from internal or vital organs to external or less vital organs and from the upper part of the body to the lower part.

The Response to the Remedy

Regarding the vital reaction which, in general terms, makes up the organism's response to the remedy, initial observers established the following guidelines borne out by time and experience:

1) An intense aggravation at the beginning of treatment, followed by a long improvement with a gradual disappearance of all problems, indicates that a good remedy has been selected.

2) A long aggravation, followed by a slight, brief improvement or no improvement at all, indicates that the case is incurable. The disease, always dynamic in its beginning, has already caused deep pathological changes which do not allow normal function to be restored. Due to a deep anatomic disturbance, there is a permanent loss of resistance in the vital organs.

3) A brief improvement, followed by an attenuated aggravation, indicates that the remedy's potency was not adequate for the case.

4) An immediate improvement without an aggravation indicates that the remedy was not well chosen and, if repeated frequently, may lead to a suppression of the symptoms as well as mask the case for future assessment.

5) A definite and prolonged improvement, without a previous aggravation and with a marked sense of wellbeing, indicates that the

exact simillimum has been prescribed, thus assuring a prolonged remission of the disease and the patient's cure.

6) Finally, in the event that the patient proves the symptoms of the prescribed remedy or successively prescribed remedies, without an amelioration of the condition, this is a case of extreme susceptibility.

The inability to reject unspecified influences indicates incurability, due to the lack of an organic will to heal.

When the homoeopath wholeheartedly accepts the philosophical principles that underpin homoeopathy, he or she can develop the perceptive abilities necessary for understanding patients and their diseases. There is no doubt that homoeopathy has the potential to deal effectively with the problem of human disease. This calls for a profound philosophical approach, penetrating into the human being's inner nature and the morbid conflict that hinders personal growth.

The Patient's Initial Improvement

Returning to the initial improvement that the patient may feel after taking a remedy, I will discuss some thoughts on the significance of disease.

When the patient reports feeling better in spite of the fact that symptoms persist, he is referring to something other than the body or the psyche. For just as we may say that the stomach is better, or the head aches, we may also say that the memory is poor, the willpower is weak, or that the intelligence is low. What is meant here is that psychological factors are as relevant to the subjective self as the stomach, head or any other part of the body. Character, the psyche and consciousness are aspects of the functioning of the individual, as real as any physical organ – although we call them mind, soul or psyche they apply as much to the self as does the dense matter of our organism.

Thus our being expresses itself as a self which fulfils its life plan as a result of the vitality that flows through soul, mind and body. We all live the unconscious reality of our innermost being, and this determines not only the complex mechanism of our will but also the energetic quality of the vital force that regulates our bodily functions. Life is a medium through which we can fully realise our potential. Disease is a struggle against the limitations of the inner and outer worlds – obstacles for the realisation of the true self.

The patient who is 'touched' by the simillimum reports feeling better, even before the mental symptoms have disappeared. He feels more in control and stronger in himself. When Hahnemann, Hering and Kent said that the patient cures himself from centre to periphery, they assigned mental symptoms to that path of cure which are nevertheless subordinate to a central self, capable of discerning sensations.

To deny the existence of this self, to which all bodily and psychological phenomena are subject, is to deny the freedom and life of which our individuality is only one expression.

Even though the phenomenon of disease is tremendously important, this does not mean we should go beyond the boundaries of practical and effective medicine. It means that we must create the conceptual values necessary for the empiric management of phenomena which medicine and psychology regard as established facts. We must bring to rational consciousness the life of our authentic selves. Only this will integrate our true personalities and enable us to become free and self-directed human beings.

Such is the fate of all individuals, well or ill, rich or poor, young or old. Disease presents itself as a complex effect of immediate or distant causes that have settled in the patient's character, symptoms and pathology.

To present the patient's problem only in terms of absolute facts, as in the case of organic, functional or psychiatric medicine, is to deny life's dynamism as a correlation of causes and effects.

The New Psychosomatic Thought

The psychosomatic trend in medicine which acknowledges the mind as directing the body is still reluctant to consider the causes that deform the life of the psyche and destroy its potential for realisation. No one can deny that psychogenic organic disorders herald a fruitful period for modern medicine. Well-known psychosomatic case studies have shown the connection between prolonged emotional conflicts and disease, such as where a nervous gastric symptom picture can bring about a peptic ulcer.

However, the crucial step has yet to be taken. The organism, with its complex psychosomatic structure, and the personality together serve a purpose which can be determined only by the innermost self that struggles to emerge to the light of consciousness.

The homoeopath is directed to the inner core of the patient. Thus, thanks to the patient's bodily self-awareness, the homoeopath can tell whether or not the prescribed remedy has stimulated the vital force in the direction of cure.

Mental and functional symptoms may persist, but the patient is better. And this perceived improvement from the depths of his being is none other than an awareness that the innermost self has been liberated.

Seen in this way, the human being has two conflicting value systems: on the one hand, disease as a physical expression of a change in the vital rhythm, inhibiting the free expression of the life force; on the other hand, the essential value of being which fulfils a specific, personal life cycle in order to develop an awareness of its own reality.

Chapter 3

Vitalism and the Law of Cure
(1966)

Before undertaking clinical practice, it is of the utmost importance to acquire firm philosophical foundations as well as a faith in homoeopathic doctrine. Many homoeopaths have failed because they thought clinical practice to be more important than an understanding of the basic principles.

In the United States, birthplace of many great masters of homoeopathy, Hahnemannian medicine declined when these masters began placing too much emphasis on the successes and failures of treated cases in their teachings, while neglecting to instil an understanding of the law of cure at work in each patient.

Constantine Hering was perhaps the best prescriber in the United States, but of the hundreds of physicians that attended his lectures, very few could follow in his footsteps. Most of them lacked his clinical perspective and thus were not as successful in their prescribing. Calvin Knerr – Hering's foremost student, who later became his son-in-law and the author of the well-known *Guiding Symptoms* – told me personally that he had never known anyone with so remarkable an intuition for prescribing a remedy as Hering. But at the same time, Knerr said, no one was as meagre in explaining how he had made his diagnosis. Hering's intuition, based on his knowledge of homoeopathic philosophy, enabled him to quickly perceive the essential symptom picture of each patient.

In the art of clinical diagnosis, as in any other applied art, there is an untransferable personal and psychological process. Science is analytical and discriminating insofar as the facts of nature are concerned, but the synthesis that links those facts depends on the researcher's ability to perceive the unity that particularises all organised beings.

This awareness allows the homoeopath to comprehend the patient's whole personality. It is the result of subconscious workings where reason and emotions come into play, yielding what has been called the clinical eye, which every practitioner with an authentic calling can and must develop. There is a general agreement on following the Hippocratic vitalist tradition. The intelligent force that coordinates vital activity and repairs damaged structures was called *enormon* by Hippocrates and *élan vital* by Bergson (1859–1941). Hahnemann fathered the law that describes its workings and the Montpellier school developed this concept philosophically, coining the term 'vital force'.

The Galenic school (Galen A.D.?131–201) has received the seal of approval of Pasteurian dogma. Seeing the germ as the essential cause of disease, the Galenic school produced several generations of materialistically minded physicians, trained to be exclusively concerned with finding and eliminating the germ, virus or toxin as the visible and specific cause of disease. What they ignored was the importance of the dynamic response of the organism in its attempt to resolve the morbid process. Unfortunately, the backward thinking that led to the rejection of the vitalist concept of disease ignored the fact that disease is not the product of some external influence or agent, but the activation of the organism's adaptive response.

Life consists of unceasing dynamic activity; that is why human beings maintain their organic and personal integrity. When faced with environmental factors such as heat, cold or humidity, or with emotional factors that threaten its integrity, the organism strives to maintain its mental and physical homoeostasis, that is to say, its wholeness as a living unit. This dynamic equilibrium is unstable, giving rise to anabolic and metabolic currents that cause the constant destruction and regeneration of cellular tissues in an endless and irreversible process. Thus, molecular changes occur in the whole organism in such a way that an individual is not the same as he was a few days ago. An ocean wave that we see coming towards us twenty metres away is not the same wave that drenches us moments later on the beach. The water molecules have transmitted motion from one to another in succession, thus forming that particular shape which we call a wave. However, millimetre by millimetre, every molecule changes on the journey. The wave has been transformed, leaving behind only a form that identifies it as such and which makes up its individuality.

It is the same with human beings. Human individuality has less to do with atoms, molecules, cells and tissues than with the activity of a structure created with a sense of life identical to the law that rules motion in the universe. Human individuality has a purpose, a vital sense that moves towards metaphysical unity. This is what makes an individual a person – not the peculiar synergy of organic functions. Nature is the perpetual transformation of never-lost electrons in cycles of contraction and dispersion that form an indistinct part of a mineral, a plant, an animal or a human being. Energy is never lost, only transformed.

Paradoxically, death is the most positive aspect of life, and metaphysically necessary, because dispersion is essential for the continuity of vital motion. What dies is the illusion of autonomy of the being that lives as an individual, without having gained awareness of his place in the totality of existence. Surely, any atom in the body has lived in another being, animal, plant, mineral or star and will continue to live in another individual after the dispersion of the body. Our death as individuals will be inevitable if we fail to fulfil the highest purpose of existence, which is to come to the realisation of cosmic unity, from which new syntheses of ever-changing forms and structures come forth. As Paracelsus (1493–1541) said, there is a complete correspondence between the microcosm and the macrocosm.

These speculations lead one to conclude that life has a meaning that can be understood by those who can perceive the law that rules the motion of cosmic energy. The law of cure that gives meaning to biological phenomena is the same law of contraction and dispersion that rules the movement of the earth and the stars and gives meaning to cosmic order. Without this absolute law in the whole of creation, there would be chaos no less in the life of a flower than in the life of a star.

The human being is creation's most perfect synthesis. A few months after birth, a human being materialises a congenital dynamic disposition which, according to Hahnemann, is of miasmatic origin. This miasm is a morbid constitutional tendency predisposing the human being to a particular pathological destiny, as yet without emotional imprints, but inevitably tending towards final dispersion or death. As humans, we grow from childish self-centredness to the psychological maturity that permits our connection with the whole and with the death of our egotistic individuality.

This progression from centre to periphery, that is, from embodiment in a living unit towards dispersion or death, is what we call the law of cure. We are born to die. Day by day, hour by hour, we use up the potential for vital energy that we bring with us at birth, as if an electric battery were being discharged. Catabolism wins over anabolism. Tissues regenerate but nevertheless harden and dry up; atheroma and conjunctive tissues replace healthy cells; skin – a kidney spread out on the body's surface – ages while eliminating waste. Like a current of energy that discharges itself from the centre, our life cycle ends with the dispersion of the elements that make up our physical body.

Even though the organism tries to counteract this disintegration, it never succeeds completely in neutralising our final deterioration or in restoring tissues to their previous state. There is never a restoration towards wholeness. There is always the organic deterioration that ends in a descent into old age and death. The purpose of the law of cure is not to prevent death, but to allow death to come smoothly and normally, thus allowing the individual to fulfil the highest purpose of existence – to become aware of his metaphysical relationship with the whole of existence.

And here we enter a philosophical terrain which is closed to science, but which must concern the physician. Does human life have a meaning, a purpose, or a knowable goal?

Yes it does, and moreover it cannot help but have one. The moral implications of the problem of chronic disease cannot be overlooked by medicine, now forced to revise the mechanistic thinking that led it to pathological dogma. The human being is not separate and autonomous, but an entity that depends on a transcendental spiritual self with a role to play in the universe. The human being develops a moral consciousness, connecting him with other human beings and with the essence of all things.

This process of personal growth takes place under the same law that regulates adaptation to the environment, organic equilibrium, inflammatory reactions and disease. The whole human being, body and mind, acts as a unit in every case of disease, coordinating the effort to restore the defences so that the individual may freely fulfil his cycle.

For example, when we have an inflammation, the congestion, local hyperthermia, immobilising pain, diapedesis, phagocytosis and abscesses, together with the fever, fear of death, accelerated heartbeat, perspiration and digestive and urinary changes, all entail a total participation of the organism under the direction of the spontaneous law of cure – leading to the outward elimination of morbid energy by expelling waste products through the skin, mucous membranes and other excretory organs. Fever is a stimulation of the processes brought into play by the organism to solve, with the appropriate temperature, any physical or emotional crisis.

Thus, in normal life as in illness, the organism employs the same resources to maintain its homoeostasis or determine its cure. These resources differ only quantitatively – in their physiological rhythm – but not in their nature. They are part of the same process, the Hippocratic *vis medicatrix naturae*, or healing power of nature. Everything happens as if an ordering intelligence acted unconsciously in the organism, to preserve it from premature dissolution as a biological unit.

Medicine must develop this concept of life in order to find that therapeutic law which also rules the motion of vital energy. When medicine considers disease to have a mere physicochemical substratum, this inevitably leads to the degeneration of the human being, by the careless suppression of the different ways in which disease seeks outward release. What materialist medicine calls disease is no more than the pathological residue of a morbid dynamism whose first expressions were suppressed with local treatments, failing to understand that what had to be cured was that very dynamic disposition.

It is in this deranged, hereditary, dynamic disposition that it is necessary to solve the problem of the miasm, that is, a *vis medicatrix* that relates to a structure damaged by past transgressions of the law of cure, and therefore insufficient in its tendency to heal. As Hahnemann pointed out, suppressing the outward releases which reflect the workings of the law of cure will have blocked the vital flow in the internal organs, thus predisposing the whole individual to premature decay. When the organism expels metabolic toxins in the form of eruptions, suppurations, diarrhoea and colds, which the liver, kidneys and glandular system have been unable to metabolise due to a diminished functional resistance, such outward releases must be respected because they indicate an attempt to protect the vital organs.

The basic problem in medicine is that of suppression – that is, blocking the fulfilment of the law of cure. All that art and science can do is rectify the vital force, so that it can cure the dynamic origin of the morbid process. Only homoeopathic remedies can do this, provided they are prescribed according to the similarity between a curative reaction experimentally produced in a healthy individual, and the natural reaction of a diseased individual, both being vital processes and expressions of the same law of cure. The fact that suppression inhibits the vital force is clear in neurotic cases, where emotional factors play an essential role.

The word 'emotion' means a moving outwards, a liberation of feelings. When emotion is repressed or sidetracked from normal consciousness, that is, from the discharge of its psychic energy, it is transformed into physical disturbances. Pathological symptoms are surrogate expressions of repressed emotions. Any physician who has reflected on the problem of human disease will agree that all pathological phenomena have a meaning – referring, in the last analysis, to impulses to action that have been repressed in either a remote or a recent past due to moral conscience.

It has been said that our civilisation's culture in regard to sex has created a punitive moral conscience provoking exaggerated depressions which can lead the human being to serious neurosis, from which he may be liberated by social movements such as existentialism, new wave, and others. I do not personally believe that such a disturbance exists in moral conscience, which I consider to be the healthiest psychological resource that the human being has. It is to moral conscience that humanity owes its spiritual evolution and the possibility of transcendence, as well as the development of religion, art, ethics and law.

What happens is that human instincts and impulses have been deranged in their dynamic origin – they have been disturbed by a miasmatic affection which compromises their functional tendency towards transforming the individual into a mature person. The cell-destroying tendencies of syphilis and sycosis make demands on the psyche which moral conscience cannot accept, thus causing it to fail. Freud maintained that this is due to an individual disposition, probably organically conditioned. Clearly, the formidable resistance of many neurotics undergoing psychoanalysis, as well as the prolonged cures necessary in most of these cases, is due to this imponderable factor which Freud called individual disposition, whose previous correction is essential.

The conscious and mature repression of sexual and aggressive instincts produces sublimation – that is, the transformation of selfish energy into impulses towards knowledge and personal development. On the other hand, instinctive suppression due to punitive coercion, not allowing emotional frustrations to be processed, determines the neurosis that Freud described as the result of the failure of repression.

The correctly chosen homoeopathic simillimum will provoke a deep curative reaction, unblocking suppressed unconscious contents and restoring the law of cure, allowing a healthy emotional concentration of psychic energy onto a single goal. A mere external treatment of symptom pictures and the elimination of crises will lead only to suppression – that is, as we have said before, to a severe transgression of the law of cure.

The physician, no matter what therapeutics he employs, must be aware that every symptom is a part of the patient's life context. Each symptom has a meaning to be unlocked, once a complete understanding has been gained of the pathological expressions and behaviour of a unique and untold human life.

Chapter 4

Mental Symptoms in Homoeopathy
(1953)

As every homoeopath knows, the character traits of a patient mirror the essence of that person's chronic disease process.

In daily practice, the physician observes that a patient's symptoms are always modified by their personality, and thus notes that symptoms are never exclusively organic. He knows from experience that emotions influence bodily functions and vice versa, but nevertheless does not necessarily have a clear understanding of this body-mind connection. The strong mechanistic influence in so much of medical training creates the habit of dissociating the psyche from the physicochemical mechanism that regulates organic functions. Ironically, even the modern psychosomatic trend in medicine has become a specialisation – as if body and psyche were two separate realities and the connection between them were not already an intrinsic part of medicine.

In Paragraph 15 of the *Organon*, Hahnemann regards the functions of the psyche as the subjective aspect of bodily functions, thus disagreeing with the Cartesian division between psyche and soma:

> The affection of the morbidly deranged, spirit-like dynamis (vital force) that animates our body in the invisible interior, and the totality of the outwardly cognizable symptoms produced by it in the organism and representing the existing malady, constitute a whole; they are one and the same. The organism is indeed the material instrument of the life, but it is not conceivable without the animation imparted to it by the instinctively perceiving and regulating dynamis, just as the vital force is not conceivable without the organism, consequently the two together constitute a unity, although in thought our mind separates this unity into two distinct conceptions for the sake of easy comprehension. (Sixth Edition, trans. Boericke)

According to Boenninghausen, the life of the psyche is an accompanying phenomenon of organic life. Soul is not separate from body. The soul gives meaning to the body and the body is the vehicle through

15

which the soul expresses itself. Psychological and organic phenomena are expressions of the same vital event.

It is from this soul, dynamis, psyche or mind, where the elements that give unity to the organism reside, that the homoeopath draws the mental symptoms that express the total reaction of the patient. But what are these mental symptoms and why do they represent the organic totality of the human being? Furthermore, what meaning do the metaphysical terms 'soul' and 'spirit' have for the modern, scientifically oriented physician?

When faced with chronic cases, the physician observes that what falls ill is undoubtedly the whole person. The diseased individual is maladjusted with respect to his environment, and expresses this conflict in the multiform language of the organs. It is necessary to understand why an individual falls ill and to discover the deep, inner meaning of their particular disease.

Human reason, a recent development in creation, is beyond our animal instincts, associative memory and practical intelligence. Thus, it is the most important organ of consciousness and confers a special meaning to the problem of disease. We may no longer say that an organism falls ill. The human being is not an organism, but has an organism that belongs to his or her being; the human being is its organism but also something more. Medicine cannot be merely biological, it is also anthropological. Anthropology is human biology – that is, biology made up of physical, mental and spiritual elements.

Because mental symptoms integrate the patient's whole symptom picture, Hahnemann assigned them the highest rank in his hierarchy of symptoms. Mental symptoms are divided into three categories: will, intelligence and memory. Of these three, the symptoms that refer to the will are ranked the highest. They are the individual's automatic reactions to organically-based impulses or sensations. They emerge from the unconscious depths of the individual, from the vital dynamism that rules over the structure, function and interconnection of tissues and organs.

The unconscious tension that we call instinct is the psychic expression of that emotional will, transmitting the requirements of cellular activity to conscious awareness. That is why organic will – the deep necessity that appears in the conscious ego as a motivation to act – is what best defines the nature of being and best summarises an individual's symptom picture.

In order to discover these symptoms of the will and, above all, in order to draw them from a patient who is perhaps unwittingly hiding the truth, or even unconsciously hostile towards us, it is necessary to know the structure of the psyche.

The symptoms we find in homoeopathic literature have been gathered from provings and transcribed with no systematisation or schematic classification. They offer no interpretation of the facts that would help us to understand the mechanism that produces them and cannot therefore be referred to any theory of the personality.

This is easily understood if Hahnemannian doctrine is considered to be purely biological. Its essential tenet is that disease is a vibratory derangement of the vital force, a dysrhythmia that disturbs the entire organism. First, physiological changes, then localised organic dysfunction and finally the structural alteration of tissues are produced. The anatomic substratum, the pathology itself, is the morphological conclusion of a process that started out as a deep shock to the vital force.

Life is an attribute of the cell, but not exclusive to each cell, because the cell cannot live separately from the organism. Life continues under other forms, in spite of the death of the cell.

At its deepest source, where the causal factors of vital dysrhythmia may be discovered, disease is intimately connected to the dynamics of the personality. Here we find it helpful to distinguish between 'personality' and the 'person'.

Personality is what we are in appearance, in terms of human relationships, what we develop in the social milieu, the mask that we build in order to face the world's demands. It is the myth that each of us lives in aspiration of the regard of others, of success and self-affirmation.

On the other hand, the person is what we are in our innermost depths. It is what conditions our moods, what we express through our unconscious will, and from where our motivations to act originate. From the depths of the person emerge thoughts and determinations which are far more powerful than what the conscious personality can ever bring forth.

Psychoanalysis is the theory that best defines these psychodynamics. Freud's division of the psyche into the conscious and the unconscious is his most valuable contribution to medical thought.

Between the body and the conscious ego there is an instinctive component of human life which has been disregarded by pathologically oriented medicine. Sydenham spoke of the existence of an invisible *homo interior* between the visible body and the mind. Corvisart (1755–1821) had said that between the physical human being and the moral human being there is always a hidden link. Freud called this instinctive or unconscious region of the mind the 'id' – that is, the cluster of

17

primary and irrational impulses, with aggression and sexual energy for its main channels.

This primitive id is ruled by pleasure. Seeking nothing else but the release of its energy through love, hate or aggression, it remains a stranger to the principles which represent worldly interests in contrast to free instinctive expression.

The ego represents the modification that the id has had to undergo when faced with the demands of the outer world. It tries to reconcile the biological, subconscious world ruled by pleasure with the objective demanding outer world. The individual must adapt to his social environment much as a live cell in a live body must adapt. This work of human and physical adaptation places the ego in constant conflict with the subconscious on the one hand and the environment on the other.

However, another region of the mind that Freud called the 'super-ego' imposes its restrictions on the id's primary impulses.

Two opposing forces then come forth in the conscious ego: on the one hand, instinctive energy and, on the other hand, the moral code implanted by parents, teachers, society, culture and religion, where spiritual values germinate and flourish.

The psyche thus consists of different aspects of a process involving the submission and absorption of instincts into more sophisticated mechanisms developed through social and spiritual life. The ego is conscious, the id is instinctive and the super-ego, which is spiritually superior, is moral conscience. These three distinct formations arise from the undifferentiated mass of impulses and tendencies that Hahnemann called the vital force, Freud called 'libido' or life instinct and Bergson called *élan vital*.

What we call 'spirit', then, is not some transcendental state of an exceptionally evolved human being, but that capacity for awareness of our own selves as subjects as well as objects within a world whose reality we must cope with.

The ego struggles with the erotic and aggressive instincts that strive to come to the conscious mind. At the same time, the ego must struggle against the feelings associated with these instincts, such as love, hate, envy, anger and resentment. If the ego is not strong enough to maintain its equilibrium, it will produce neurotic symptoms that are the different compromising strategies which the ego employs to protect itself from such instincts.

The physician must therefore be attuned to this process of the personality which, to a greater or lesser extent, every patient will express. The homoeopath works with the symptoms that the patient translates through a compromised ego, 'falsified', so to speak, by those very compromises destined to defend it from his instincts and the punitive censorship of the super-ego. This makes it difficult to draw out the patient's mental symptoms. More than just hearing about them, the homoeopath must try to 'see' them and interpret them through and in spite of the patient's ego.

Anguish, anxiety, fear, phobias and obsessions are the products of that insecurity and sense of risk with which the ego lives as it struggles between instinctive impulses and the demands of the super-ego.

One kind of defence mechanism that the ego sets up to protect itself from these impulses is repression, often causing much anguish in which the patient is completely unaware of his instincts. Another is conversion hysteria, in which a patient's conflicts with his or her instincts settle in one or more organs, leading to physical symptoms.

Other common defence mechanisms are compensatory responses. For example, amiable, kind, altruistic, moralistic, religious, arrogant, proud, sarcastic or derisive attitudes will tend to mask the exact opposite feelings.

Patients may also project on to another person the rejection, resentment or guilt that they themselves feel for others, thus feeling rejected, offended or humiliated by others.

In Lachesis, for instance, we see projection in a characteristic symptom – jealousy. A patient going through the menopause may feel jealousy without knowing it. Rejecting her sexual desires from her conscious mind, Lachesis projects this exacerbated stimulus on to her spouse, whom she accuses of being unfaithful.

These and other defence mechanisms such as regression or isolation are effective neurotic ways by which patients can protect themselves from their basic impulses. Defence mechanisms are fixed in a patient's character as traits which the homoeopath must thoroughly scrutinise – not only do they consume a great deal of the patient's energy, thus undermining his enjoyment of work and life, but they also tend to alter the objective truth concerning the patient's condition. Not surprisingly, there are patients who do not want to get cured, who unconsciously prefer to continue to be ill, because their illness shields them from destructive or dangerous impulses. In this way, their guilt feelings and the need for self-punishment which their super-ego demands of them are assuaged.

One patient had all the physical but none of the mental characteristics of Natrum Muriaticum. In fact, her mental symptoms were the exact opposite of Natrum Muriaticum's. She was especially kind and submissive to her husband. Furthermore, she assured me that she could not bear to be separated from him for a moment, that his love filled her with joy and happiness, that she enjoyed being with people and that she responded well to praise and affection. The very emphasis with which she spoke was suspect and she actually ended the interview in tears. The best case-taking is done when patients are allowed to speak for themselves.

As in the Natrum Muriaticum case, another patient had all the Lycopodium physical symptoms but none of the mental ones. His active, optimistic, confident, patient, good-humoured, extroverted and arrogant personality was a cover for a deep feeling of inferiority, which he struggled against and tried to hide.

Thus, in order to discover what is behind a patient's mental symptoms, it is essential for the homoeopath to be familiar with the various defence mechanisms that an individual may employ.

From the depths of vitality in the human being rise currents of energy that seek release throughout the whole organism, from the centre to the periphery, from the more vital organs to the less vital organs, from the mind to the excretory organs.

Mind and body behave in the same way. Freud's libido follows a path from centre to periphery that entails the same psychic release that Hahnemann's vital force fulfils when internal processes surface and toxins are eliminated. Like Plato's Eros and Bergson's *élan vital*, both libido and vital force are the same centrifugal current of energy that travels the path to final biological disintegration.

When this free outward flow of vital energy is blocked, the initial stages of disease are produced. Hahnemann called this 'psora', which is the basic disorder conditioned by suppression in all its forms. The word emotion comes from the Latin *emovere*, which means 'to come out', and expresses the physical release of erotic and aggressive feelings through all organs, in the same way that morbid products are eliminated. As Hahnemann maintained, cure is brought about from the mind to the organs. For example, when a tuberculosis patient suffers from mental symptoms, his pulmonary symptoms disappear. On the other hand, unless the mental symptoms improve, the pulmonary symptoms will not only recur but will be aggravated. Hahnemann considered mental metastasis to be the deepest and most entrenched stage of the morbid process.

Depth psychology is familiar with the correlation between the emotions and the organs through which they seek expression. Thus, anguish expresses itself through the heart and the lungs, fear through the thyroid glands, disgust through the bile, anger through the encephalic arteries, avarice through the intestines, greed through the stomach, sexuality through the genital organs and the heart, and so on. Kent maintained that these correspondences have pragmatic value within the law of similars.

The skilled homoeopath knows that if a patient's gastrointestinal symptoms improve, but the mental symptoms worsen, the order of cure has been inverted and therefore the prescription must be antidoted.

When aggressive, destructive or death instincts arise from a patient's organic depths and prevail over erotic or life instincts, it is because the patient is suffering in the very core of their being. The whole system is deeply disturbed, and this is expressed through mental symptoms such as hate, suicidal and criminal tendencies, aversion to people, including children, indifference, resentment, fear and anxiety.

These are the symptoms that reveal the morbid spirit of a patient and it is the homoeopath's task to discover them through the suffering personality that appears in the consulting room.

Chapter 5

Unicism and Pluralism
(1959)

Real progress in homoeopathy is attained when homoeopaths perfect their skills in choosing the correct single remedy.

Every patient's dynamis has a unique way of conditioning his particular morbid process. People are not ill because they have a disease; they have a disease because they are ill. A basic tenet since Hahnemann's time is to take note of each patient's individual symptoms and match them with tried and proven remedies – repeated remedy provings have yielded constant psychological and sensory reactions. This Hahnemannian approach is in line with ancient Hippocratic thought and has not been surpassed by any of the dissident homoeopathic tendencies which prescribe several remedies at one time in order to address certain symptoms, partial syndromes or even organic lesions, without regarding the whole patient.

The homoeopathic law of similars is correlated to the guideline that Hahnemann establishes in Paragraph 3 of his *Organon* concerning the holistic approach in medicine. In order to know precisely what is to be treated in each case, the physician must have something more than a knowledge of therapeutics; he must also have a profound knowledge of chronic and acute disease. The division among unicists, pluralists and those who advocate combination remedies stems from the idea each group has of what must be cured in each case. If the physician has a pathological, organic concept of disease, it is only natural that he may wish to cure what he has diagnosed as the affected organ. Pluralists tend to divide the organism into different levels that react differently to different remedies; thus, pluralists usually prescribe a constitutional remedy, a remedy for localised symptoms and a remedy to stimulate the eliminating function of an organ – all in the name of the practice of drainage.

However, the diseased organ is not the disease. Toxins and tissue damage are only a by-product of the real disease which is, in turn, a result of a dynamic derangement of the whole organism. As the

Hippocratic aphorism says: 'Man is but an organ, the organism but a function.' The individualisation that homoeopathic diagnosis requires is a task that is at once singular and holistic.

Hahnemann established as a basic clinical principle the unity of the patient's reaction: that is, the totality of symptoms that reflect the dynamic derangement. This very personal total symptom picture can never be the expression of an affected isolated organ or a disturbed localised function.

To prescribe a homoeopathic remedy in terms of a partial number of localised symptoms, without taking into account the individual's mental and physical traits, is to suppress symptoms and reject the Hippocratic *vis medicatrix*. The law of cure is fulfilled only by acting on the dynamic core of the disease process, which is not revealed through laboratory tests or physical signs but only through the characteristic symptoms of the patient's complete history.

Nevertheless, in the case of adult patients, it is true that the physician must inevitably base the diagnosis on the totality of the patient's most recent symptoms. This is what determines the prescription for an acute episode or for the patient's current disease. Therefore it is only a similar remedy and not the simillimum corresponding to the patient's whole, constitutional symptom picture. The simillimum may be employed in the first prescription for adults without any serious pathological lesions and is generally indicated for children.

In infancy, the single remedy is easily identifiable. The stress of life, with its many transgressions of natural laws, plus the infections we have contracted, tends to mask our pure, original, constitutional symptom picture. As we go through life we accumulate spurious symptoms that are the result of our personal lifestyles. These, however, are often cured by better hygiene, a more natural diet and a lifestyle in harmony with our moral principles. Without using any remedies whatsoever, this is precisely what psychoanalytic cures accomplish: they restore the autonomy of a self compelled by instinct and conscience to waver between hysterical perversions and obsessive guilt feelings.

If a patient has mental but no physical symptoms, he will probably respond well to psychotherapy. In order to prescribe a homoeopathic remedy, it is necessary to obtain a complete mental and physical symptom picture. But even if the remedy similar to the secondary symptom picture produced by infections, toxins or personality disorders is prescribed, it is still necessary to diagnose according to the latent characteristic syndrome that predisposed the patient to infections or neurosis in the first place. We arrive, then, at the goal of true therapeutics: the constitutional predisposition that moulds the individual's character and vital reaction to the process of adaptation.

Hahnemann clearly stated the need to find the patient's simillimum when he or she has suffered a relapse of symptoms after the most recent prescription. In any case, symptoms are the only intelligible expression of the organism's dynamic derangement. Whether to identify the remedy similar to the current acute symptom picture or to the constitutional simillimum, our only true guide is a complete history of symptoms, faithfully translated into the language of the repertory. We say 'faithfully translated', because symptoms are not a mere transcription of what the patient says, but a correct translation of all observable data.

One 11-year-old patient, according to his mother, was excessively orderly and meticulous. He carried out a nightly ritual before going to bed, laying out, adjusting and readjusting his bedclothes to the centimetre. He also tore up his notebooks because he thought that his homework was never properly done. In Kent's *Repertory* we find two clearly defined mental symptoms that corresponded to this boy's obsessiveness: 'Conscientious about trifles' and 'Irresolution'. These symptoms, when linked to his general symptoms, yielded a perfect Silica picture that otherwise would not have been evident unless his mental symptoms had been interpreted.

As we have said before, toxins and damaged tissues and organs are not the disease but the result of a dynamic disease process, and cannot therefore guide the homoeopath to the diagnosis and prescription. Drainage is not based on symptoms but on the action that remedies exert on certain organs, as in Chelidonium for the liver, Hepar Sulphuris for suppurations, Pulsatilla for mucous membranes, Berberis for the kidneys, Ceanothus for the spleen, and so on. This approach does not take symptom analogies into account and repeats the error of confusing the lesion with the disease itself. We do not take issue with the validity of prescribing draining remedies chosen for their action on organs or tissues – the whole drug is based on the need to favour the organism's eliminating function (as in purging remedies, ulcerations, diuretics and so on, advocated by Hippocrates and Paracelsus). However, before and after prescribing draining remedies or remedies with local action, the physician must address the dysfunction of the individual that generated the toxins and pathology in the first place. This is only possible by detecting the patient's characteristic symptoms.

If the physician can identify the single active remedy that corresponds to the patient's particular morbid predisposition, and if the patient does not have irreversible tissue damage, cure will be brought about from the centre to the periphery with no need of drainage. This is not speculation or esoteric medical doctrine, but a verifiable, everyday clinical reality. Both orthodox medicine and organ-based homoeopathy take only pathological consequences into account, disregarding the patient's dynamic constitutional aetiology. The problem of mental and physical disease treated by this approach cries out for a solution.

The practice of drainage and also organ-based therapies such as nutrition, physiotherapy, surgery and psychiatry make sense if they support the clinical concept of the unique pathogenic dynamism present in each individual patient. If the physician has actually interrogated the patient and not just examined that patient's organism, then he will have the necessary guidelines to know how to stimulate the *vis medicatrix*.

Polypharmacy causes much confusion both in homoeopathy and in conventional medicine. In Paragraph 273 of the *Organon* Hahnemann states: 'In no case under treatment is it necessary and *therefore not permissible* to administer to a patient more than *one single, simple medicinal* substance at a time.' He goes on to say in Paragraph 274: 'As the true physician finds in simple medicines, administered singly and uncombined, all that he can possibly desire ... he will, mindful of the wise maxim that "it is wrong to attempt to employ complex means when simple means suffice", never think of giving as a remedy any but a single, simple medicinal substance.'

It is anti-homoeopathic to prescribe a remedy that does not correspond to the patient's characteristic symptoms. Just as a patient cannot have two diseases at the same time, he can never have two or more characteristic groups of symptoms. Moreover, further clinical interpretation of the symptoms that arise after the first dose will never be possible if several remedies are prescribed at the same time, because their simultaneous effects are impossible to register separately. The curative effect does not consist in merely knowing that the patient has improved, but in activating the law of cure. When prescribing a well-chosen remedy, it is possible to foresee which symptoms will reappear and which ones will disappear.

Homoeopathy is empirically applied. To expect a patient's response to a prescribed remedy only in terms of a mere improvement or the disappearance of symptoms does not make it a rational form of therapeutics.

The homoeopathic remedy acts on the deep dynamic cause of disease. With great genius, Hahnemann established the three main miasms of psora, syphilis and sycosis, which correspond to the three physiological modes of cellular activity: excitation, inhibition and perversion. There is always a dynamic terrain that provides the conditions for infections, intoxications, traumas, deficiencies and mental disturbances. Thus it is mistaken to believe that the homoeopathic remedy is a symptomatic remedy. Basing its diagnosis on the patient's most recent characteristic symptom picture, homoeopathy does not suppress symptoms but modifies their miasmatic origin.

By adhering to dynamic symptom analogies and not speculative diagnoses or tissue damage, the homoeopath will be seeking the single remedy with whose pathogenesis he is familiar. This will not only allow the law of cure to be observed, but will also enhance his knowledge of materia medica – the goal of every homoeopath. Pluralism claims to be right by virtue of the success it has in the eyes of the general public, but pluralists also recognise that these successes are uncontrollable in their outcome. When based on a thorough knowledge of the patient's symptoms, the well-chosen single remedy will activate the law of cure in all the physiological planes in which vital activity is supposedly divided, and will follow a recognised and predictable path.

Pluralists prescribe two or more remedies at the same time, to be taken alternately or serially, contending that each remedy applies to one symptom or one part of the symptoms of the disease. In doing so, they apply the law of coexistence, which is undoubtedly a true law. However, because the law of similars aims for the total rather than the partial recovery of the individual, it refers to the patient's characteristic totality – that is to say, his or her whole mental and physical symptom picture. Individuality entails unity and indivisibility. Therefore, there cannot be more than one single remedy with the same dynamic action, even though the localised organic symptoms that it can produce in provings may well vary from subject to subject.

Remedy provings have been carried out on many different types of constitutions; thus it will not be possible for each prover to reproduce exactly all the symptoms generated by one single remedy. By the same token, it is equally impossible for a specific remedy with a specific action to account for all the morbid phenomena that one particular individual may have. If the homoeopath takes note only of localised organic symptoms, he will naturally find syndromes that correspond to different remedies. On the other hand, if he takes into account the numerical totality of symptoms, he may find the diversity that belongs to all natural phenomena, but will fail to see the essential unity that rules dynamic vitality as the supreme destiny of every human being: that is, evolution into maturity.

Medicine must seek this essential goal of health and fulfil the law of cure. Only thus will medicine enable human beings to exhaust the karma of their disease and evolve towards the psychological maturity that will connect them with values of transcendence and freedom. If not, physicians remain unaware of their true mission, and of what to cure in each case. But if the goal is only to palliate by suppressing symptoms through a pathological approach, the physician may apply several remedies simultaneously for the various consequences of vital phenomena, disregarding their dynamic origin. The practice of medicine very much depends on each physician's ideals and values and on his or her level of maturity.

Personally, I would have more faith in the physician who subscribes both to mechanistic rationalism and finalist vitalism, and aspires to connect with life's transcendental values. This physician would not only have an intellectual conception of the human being, but would also perceive the cosmic unity of humanity with its environment, and have insight into the various centres that regulate complex vital activity. From the time of Hippocrates until today, mechanistic, analytical thought has prevailed over the vitalist teachings of Paracelsus, Haehl, Hahnemann and others. Because the soul directs and regulates the body, the disturbances it suffers generate disease and pathology.

We do not deny the success that the application of various remedies combined in a complex may have. Neither do we deny the success that several remedies taken successively at hourly, daily or even weekly intervals may have, or the success that remedies prescribed on the basis of iridology, fingernail analysis or an abstract disease diagnosis may also have. Any therapeutic method may be effective. Physicians may inspire confidence in patients who may be especially receptive. Or perhaps, among the various homoeopathic remedies, some of them eradicate certain groups of symptoms and this satisfies the patient temporarily. But, from experience and on principle, we know that this success is uncertain and inconsistent because the patient is still ill, albeit in another form, even though he or she may always remember with gratitude the homoeopath who 'got rid of' his headaches, lumbago or other ailments.

No conscientious physician can delude himself regarding so-called 'cures' that do not come from rational therapeutic principles, nor from homoeopathy in the true sense of the word. Furthermore, there will always be opportunists who have scant knowledge of the discipline, little confidence in their remedies, and a belief that disease can be treated locally while disregarding the patient's whole life context, and who make a prescription without taking the time to select an individual remedy with care. They are the ones who accuse homoeopathy of being imperfect – because it does not solve the problem of their lack of expertise in 'taking the case' without the effort, dedication and training that this requires.

In spite of everything that has been published in order to make it easier for the homoeopath to find the simillimum more rapidly, difficulties usually arise when searching for the constitutional remedy. Hunches, impressions or intuitions do not take the place of careful symptom analysis. The homoeopath must identify the characteristics that single out the patient's dynamic derangement – that is, his constitutional predisposition to structure a determined pathology. The apparent disease is not a cause but an effect of the real disease that has constituted the patient's characteristic personality, habits and ailments. The patient's underlying diathesis or morbid predisposition is not discovered merely by observing symptoms of organic malfunction or disturbed mechanisms, but by appreciating the integral functioning of a whole person in their adaptation to life.

Syphilitic, tubercular or sycotic stigma will pervert the individual's instinctiveness, leading in turn to the psychological conflict that disturbs his life and, consequently, to the formation of a pathological lesion. No matter what the therapeutic orientation of the physician may be, the state of the psyche and moral conduct are the psychological connotation of the physical problem. In order to attain a cure, the physician must refer the physiopathological mechanisms directly to their main cause, which resides in the mental state. And it is there, in the patient's mental symptoms, that we may find the unique, peculiar traits that determine his or her individuality. This mental symptom picture has a composition similar to one single remedy.

Aside from this, the physician who ponders an individual's life history must know whether that person has oriented his life in a positive and creative way. In other words, the physician must determine whether the patient's actions favour a constructive participation in the community as a mature individual.

The homoeopathic concept of disease as a vital defensive reaction supports Hering's dynamic law of cure, from the vital centres of the individual to the excretory periphery. However, it must be noted that this law not only concerns the centrifugal path through which toxins are eliminated, but more importantly that it also controls the evolution of the subject towards psychological health. No matter what is valued in different cultures, health in this case implies overcoming dependent self-centredness and growing into morally responsible adults. Health is not attained if a patient continues to be stuck in regressive behaviour patterns, unresolved resentments and frustrations.

Inevitably, this synthetic vision of the clinical symptom picture is the result of a deep perception of chronic disease. When the physician aims to understand the patient's whole history, he will arrive at the constitutional diathesis that generated the current pathological process. There is no such thing as a localised disease in which the whole organism as a biological unit is not involved. However, in clinical practice this holistic approach must include non-mechanical factors which organic medicine cannot comprehend because they lie beyond the frontier of experimental science. We refer to those mental symptoms that stand out with regard to ethical values and which make homoeopathy a humanistic medical practice.

Undoubtedly, in the process of mental life and in the human personality there are extraphysical factors that make the psyche impossible to scrutinise, let alone interpret, in terms of current mechanistic science. However, thanks to experimentation with infinitesimal doses of potentised substances in healthy individuals, it has been possible to expose deeply buried mental phenomena and experiences related to ethics and human values. Homoeopathy has made it possible to integrate these values into clinical practice as valuable scientific data, in order to obtain an individualised, pathological symptom picture.

Far from being burdensome, it is a spiritual delight for the homoeopath who, imbued with the principles expounded by Hahnemann in his *Organon*, aims to draw the distinctive character traits from the patient's clinical history.

Chapter 6

Which School of Homoeopathy?
(1964)

As is widely acknowledged, there are two schools of homoeopathy, each differing in their teachings and approach. One school considers disease as a mechanism by which physical and chemical alterations and tissue lesions express themselves as classifiable syndromes. Its method of cure is oriented towards correcting the diagnosed malfunction or lesion. Regardless of the pathogenic interpretation, remedy prescriptions according to this school are entirely based on localised symptoms, whether they are of an affected organ or a disturbed system. Because the whole patient has not been taken into account, it makes little difference whether conventional or homoeopathic remedies are prescribed. The homoeopath who prescribes Apis to treat an oedema as if it were an isolated symptom is using the same approach as an orthodox physician who prescribes a diuretic. Both make the greatest transgression that is possible in medicine – to suppress symptoms without curing the patient.

The other school considers disease as a deep vibratory disturbance of the vital principle or spiritual energy that animates the physical body. Because all biological strata are affected, the body's integrity as a functioning unit is compromised. Moreover, this derangement has a meaning: it is organic behaviour that reflects the nature of the patient's total morbid dynamics, indicating what must be cured in each individual.

This school of homoeopathy, imbued in Hahnemannian thought, formulates principles and laws of vital activity which rule over the process of disease and cure, and which no physician who has a calling for truth may reject.

Thus we may conceive of a common link among the many currents of medical thought. Each with their own peculiar way of becoming ill, patients will consult any physician, no matter what school he or she belongs to, with the sole purpose of being helped and understood.

Indeed, the conceptual and ethical antagonism between both schools is the same antagonism that exists between good and bad medical practice. While one school employs polypharmacy, combination medicines or serially prescribed remedies in order to address pathological symptoms, the other school strives to address the patient's entire symptom picture in an integral manner, prescribing the only possible single remedy adequate for the present moment. While one school palliates symptoms in order to please the client, the other school is committed to gaining an intimate and sympathetic understanding of the patient, in order to enhance effectively his or her *vis medicatrix*.

Vitalist Hippocratic medicine acknowledges the undoubtedly valuable contribution of experimental medicine in the exploration of the physiopathological mechanism, but it also emphasises the dynamic derangement of that coordinating principle which Claude Bernard (1813–78) referred to as the decisive factor in the morbid process.

Homoeopath or not, the physician who thinks and acts accordingly, is closer to true homoeopathy than the homoeopath who advocates polypharmacy and combination medicines. These homoeopaths fail to understand the damage caused by suppressive medicine obstructing the organism's eliminating functions, which are the by-product of chronic disease.

For those orthodox colleagues who condemn homoeopathy, we will defend two basic premises: in the first place, the homoeopath is not a combatant who tries to 'annihilate' disease, but a collaborator who aims actively to help disease, perceiving it as a dynamic reaction whose nature is to restore homoeostasis, even though it is not capable of attaining this purpose by itself. To borrow a phrase from von Weizsäcker, the homoeopathic remedy tells the vital force: 'Yes, but not in that way!'

In the second place, as for those who think that homoeopathy is based on suggestion, we will say that the subject in homoeopathy has a different meaning from what it has in psychoanalysis or in psychosomatic medicine. Moreover, homoeopathy does not have its own psychology. If it is true that, in homoeopathy, mental symptoms define the patient's morbid process, it is nevertheless also true that they are the product, as are all other reactions and sensations, of remedy provings. Mental symptoms are not the result of deductive or theoretical speculations, but the faithful transcription of what the subject who is under the effects of a potentised remedy feels, perceives or expresses as personality or emotional reactions.

We strongly wish to demonstrate that when correctly and responsibly practised, homoeopathy is not a therapy of suggestion, nor an esoteric doctrine, but a legitimate medical discipline.

Chapter 7

Mental Symptoms and the Meaning of 'Totality' in Homoeopathy
(1957)

With the advent of Hahnemannian homoeopathy at the beginning of the nineteenth century, the ancient Hippocratic concept of 'totality' was again brought to the forefront. To perceive the whole patient was once again an essential clinical objective. Thus medicine had the opportunity of complying with the precept supported by all the great masters of clinical practice, that disease can be understood only in terms of the whole human being.

Nevertheless, validated by discoveries in physiology, bacteriology and biochemistry, organic medicine segregated the pathological lesion from the patient and began to study the isolated organ, divorced from the patient's whole life context. Absorbed by this scientific endeavour, organic medicine overlooked the fact that the lesion is not the cause of disease but only its consequence. Disease is the result of a dynamic process, of an alteration of organic functions that compromise the totality of each individual. Some homoeopaths, trained according to the principle that the pathological lesion and organic disease are products of a vital derangement involving the whole individual in a single total reaction, have lost this tenet of Hahnemannian doctrine and have committed themselves to symptomatic medicine, giving no thought to wholeness. It is an urgent task to restore this principle of wholeness.

Above all, it is necessary to clarify a basic principle that gives meaning to a homoeopath's clinical practice. The patient who consults a physician is subject to a detailed scrutiny of his most recent symptoms. This individualisation of the case leads to the selection of a remedy that matches the patient's particular current syndrome, which, according to Hahnemann, corresponds to the currently activated miasm. However, this type of diagnosis is precarious.

The current ailment, together with the total physical and psychological reaction experienced in the present moment, expresses an underlying constitutional chronic process which has conditioned the emergence of the current symptom picture. Homoeopathy is sidetracked from its real task if it is content with prescribing for the current symptom picture and neglects to inquire into the morbid constitutional terrain that has predetermined the current ailment.

The main objective of Hahnemannian homoeopathy is to match the individualisation of the remedy similar to the current symptom picture with the individualisation of the constitutional remedy, which is the true simillimum of the case. The dynamic action of the constitutional remedy must coincide with the morbid spirit of the patient's dynamic core: that is, with his or her deep-seated personality.

If Hahnemann had not begun the *Organon* by stating that the only mission of the physician is to cure, and if he had not maintained in Paragraph 3 that the physician must know 'what is to be cured ... in every individual case of disease' as well as 'what is curative in medicines', the practice of homoeopathy would have been reduced to the local application of remedies more or less similar to the patient's current needs.

But this was not what Hahnemann had in mind. His study of the miasms as the dynamic substratum of chronic disease has undoubtedly provided insight into the constitutional problem, but at the same time has also compelled the homoeopath to have more honesty and intelligence in the analysis of each individual case.

Ever since Hahnemann wrote the *Organon*, no homoeopath is exempt from the obligation to transcribe a complete clinical history. This will help the physician relate the nature of the patient's current symptom picture to that person's personal life history. The physician's *leitmotif* is to discover the key to the patient's illness. This key to the case reflects the patient's characteristic mood, conflicts of adaptation and morbid constitutional terrain. As Hahnemann maintained, no remedy is the simillimum unless it contains the patient's mental character or spirit.

Functional disturbances of the organism and local alterations must be referred to the totality of the patient's symptoms – the totality of symptoms reflects the patient's soul. General symptoms and organic sensations depend on the patient's personality structure. As Claude Bernard maintained, 'The vital force directs phenomena that it does not produce, in contrast to the physical agent that produces phenomena that it does not direct.' (*Les liquides de l'organisme*, Vol. 3, 1839)

The totality of symptoms that reflect the patient's chronic disease is neither any single one of those symptoms, nor the sum of all of them. Just as a melody or a musical chord is something new and different from the individual tones of which it is composed, something new has emerged from the harmonious integration of symptoms.

The experimental psychology of the nineteenth century aimed to construct a picture of the human personality by measuring and combining the various individual psychic functions. It was only with the advent of holistic psychology that personality began to be considered not as a mere composite of separate experiences, but as the total reaction of a living being, distinct from each and every sensation. Similarly, in current medicine, the system is conceived as a 'summary' of the complex interaction of diencephalic regulatory centres, where essential elements of the personality come together with the physical and biochemical systems as functional categories. Peripheral regulation and events in the organic visceral zone also depend upon the oscillations of biological 'will' originating from diencephalic centres which act as a central coordinating isthmus of the personality.

In the study of each patient, the physical, organic, psychic and environmental factors must be integrated into a clinical synthesis which allows the physician to view the case with a morbid tendency and destiny that is valid for that individual.

When von Bergmann (1836–1907), who created functional pathology, studied gastroduodenal ulcers he observed that the ulcerous lesion was not the cause of the disease, but a disorder due to a constitutional stigma rooted in the patient's bodily and mental terrain.

This anthropological insight has helped the physician understand that the task is not to describe the morbid process but to discover the importance that this process has for the patient, and what role it plays in his or her whole life and what it means to be cured. No valid prognosis can be based exclusively on organic processes – time and again, physicians have observed patients with a fatal prognosis survive, as they have a strong will to live which counteracts the natural tendency to final dispersion or self-destruction.

We do not know if science will some day measure this will to live, this Hippocratic *physis*, *natura medicatrix* or immanent principle of biological activity that propels the human being towards growth, evolution and freedom. However, we do know that if a person's will to heal is not stimulated, whether spontaneously, or with a dynamic form of therapeutics or by any other means, the law of cure, which is his preservation and destiny, will not be activated.

This is what Hahnemann clearly states in Paragraph 3 of the *Organon* and what he develops in his concept of chronic disease. To perceive the clinical case requires that the diagnostic value of symptoms be conferred by the understanding of the patient's whole and unique life history. The research supplied by physics, chemistry and biology allows the physician to gather the data into a harmonious whole and give birth to the clinical reality of the case. This is what Hahnemann establishes when he says in Paragraph 153 that the physician must take into account only 'the more striking, singular, uncommon and peculiar signs and symptoms of the case of disease … for it is more particularly these that very similar ones in the list of symptoms of the selected medicine must correspond to …' A natural cure will never be brought about unless mental and emotional symptoms are addressed.

One of the most difficult paradoxes is that of patients who have eradicated their disease, have corrected their pathology and have improved their symptoms, but nevertheless are mentally and emotion-ally worse, and less able to deal with their circumstances. The inner-most core has remained untouched, or even worsened. Sooner or later, the physician realises that he has treated the products of the disease but not the disease itself. Thus, from a Hahnemannian perspective, what must be cured in these circumstances is the mood, character or vital attitude of the patient towards life.

Undoubtedly, medication that solves the patient's immediate prob--lem complies with the patient's momentary requirements – often the patient asks for no more than this. Patients do not usually know what it is that must be cured in them, but ask the physician to restore a balance in their emotional and mental life that they think depends on their organic ailment. To treat a patient for diabetes, rheumatism, a stomach ulcer, an inflamed gallbladder or any other organic ailment does not solve the patient's essential pathological problem. To attend to these localised affections can, however, restore a relative balance which may be mistaken for a real cure. This, in fact, is what occurs in many cases where the patient attains some degree of physical and mental health. Here the physician who really knows the patient is aware that he must not 'touch' the constitutional substratum, must not stir the latent diathesis that will muddy the still waters of a precarious but effective homoeostasis.

Human beings are healthy when they fulfil the purpose of their existence. If it is true that the physician must reach the level of spiritual determination in order to do something more, he also relies on the patient's will to heal, which is often simply not there. In chronic diseases, the patient's psychic reaction generates a functional patho-logical syndrome which provides feedback to the organism's response. This explains why addressing the current pathological problem always improves the patient and often cures, by suppressing the retrograde influx of the organic lesion on the nervous system. The Hippocratic statement that there are no diseases, but only diseased people, may be modified by saying that there are both diseases and diseased people.

According to Hahnemann, the so-called mental and emotional diseases are only organic diseases in which mental disturbances are aggravated while physical symptoms diminish. Because Hahnemann does not accept that there is an autonomous psychic life separate from bodily processes, he considers neurosis as a functional derangement of the whole person. Neurosis and physical disease are concomitant functions of a disease process that begins with a disturbance in emotional development.

Neurosis is not a separate chapter of medical practice, nor a phenomenon of functional pathology. Because the organism is an active individuality which needs to adapt to its environment and maintain its homoeostasis, it must respond to circumstances with a behaviour adequate to its internal needs. The processes through which the human being experiences his needs or organic states are the psychic processes that include sensations, experiences and emotions, as well as perception, imagination, memory, intuition and intelligence. Organically conditioned behaviour is inclined towards the individual's functional wellbeing, and therefore the sensations of heat, cold, hunger, sadness and so on propel him towards a broad range of attitudes that tend to satisfy his need to protect himself from difficulties. The general and characteristic symptoms in homoeopathy are the same mental symptoms that direct the individual's behaviour. When faced with changes in temperature, the need for food, or sensory impressions, impulses and feelings, the human being will respond by developing the appropriate defence mechanisms or means of adaptation.

The human being is biologically open to the environment, thus developing a process of unfolding his biological and psychological needs, which are synthesised into what we may call a vital attitude. This vital attitude of adaptation is expressed through the complex set of organic symptoms, sensations, perceptions and emotional reactions which come together to preserve the basic instinct of conservation – that is, the will to live, to assert oneself freely and protect one's individuality. The obstacles to this self-determination are those which, due to the interplay between a faulty constitution of miasmatic origin and adverse external factors, make up the personal 'key' of the morbid process.

No single symptom, syndrome or sign of a disease, no matter how striking it may seem in the patient, can by itself determine a diagnosis. Only a synthesis with a realistic anthropological criterion allows the physician to understand the derangement in the core of the patient, from where all symptoms of biological will arise – which Hahnemann ranked as essentially characteristic symptoms. Here lies the key to the patient's mistaken vital attitude. This is the synthesis that the physician has to create in order to know what must be treated and cured.

The human being has vital, emotional and spiritual needs which overlap each other in order to express the activity of the vital force. Whether or not we are vitalists in medicine, we must acknowledge that the human being is a dynamic entity driven by the 'breath of life', progressing through different stages of psychic development and following a centrifugal path from childish self-centredness to the opening of the self to transcendent reality.

Disease comes from the obstruction of this evolving process which motivates human beings towards responsibility and full consciousness. The patient's current symptom picture of pathology, pains, spasms, sensations and mental symptoms is an expression of a primary derangement of the vital force considered as biological will: disposition, anxiety, appetite, passion, libido or, in scientific terms, a stimulus that flows from the physical body to the psyche, thus becoming instinct. When this vital stimulus suffers repression from an opposing environment and culture, an intense stress is produced, which Hahnemann called psora.

Under the action of the homoeopathic remedy, long-buried unconscious feelings such as jealousy, envy, fear and anguish are stirred. Old childhood memories are relived; sensations and attitudes that were thought to be outgrown come to the fore. Current mental symptoms, as derived from the patient's case history, are usually the product of the defence mechanisms that hide the patient's true constitutional nature.

Resentment, envy, aggression, destructiveness and guilt feelings which overwhelm the adult today are the result of feelings of anguish brought on by the negative judgments of parents and elders that generated the sensation of being bad, ugly or dull in the child of yesterday.

With a clinical sense of what is characteristic and significant in the patient, and grounded in a profound knowledge of the human soul – as Hahnemann requires – the homoeopath can perceive the patient's vital attitude towards life. With the remedy that matches the current symptom picture, the physician stirs repressed unconscious feelings. The patient's true constitutional symptoms may then surface, enabling the true simillimum to be found, if it should differ from the remedy prescribed for the current or most recent symptom picture.

No matter what clinical category the patient belongs to, whether organic, lesional, functional, neurotic or psychotic, the personal background must be studied, not only regarding the circumstances which have brought about the current symptom picture but also the vital attitude, thus conferring meaning to the entire morbid process.

Chapter 8

Curing the Constitutional Disease
(1969)

Medicine's age-old quest has been to discover the individual's general inclination or disposition to disease. It has always sought broad general principles that would allow a better understanding of the dynamic and prepathological nature of disease, that is, the basic tendency towards certain clinical expressions. It is a question of understanding the constitutional predisposition to a particular vital attitude and organic pathology.

There seems to be a basic philosophical agreement, whether in ancient oriental thought or in modern western conjectures, on the existence of a primitive biological consciousness in the human being which links diseases with the development of the personality.

The study of the human mind has been the most perplexing concern of medicine of all time. It is no longer strange to acknowledge that organic and psychosomatic ailments, such as tuberculosis and cancer, do not arise without a disturbance of the personality. The ancient Hippocratic theory of the four humours or temperaments – choleric, sanguine, phlegmatic and bilious – assigned a special clinical category to the character of each temperament. Melancholy, for example, corresponded to affections of the spleen, hypochondria and anxiety about health to affections of the liver. Thus Hippocrates laid down the original foundations of psychosomatic medicine.

The analytic approach that has characterised medical research since the nineteenth century has focused its attention mainly on the aetiology and symptomatology of diseases, overlooking disease as a whole. This approach entails a metaphysical pitfall which, ironically, is tacitly forbidden by scientific materialism.

The Pasteurian germ theory was a great scientific contribution to the knowledge of certain diseases. However, dazzled by the possibility of therapeutic access to the specific germ, conventional medicine went far beyond Pasteur's own conclusions. Towards the end of his life, he maintained that the terrain is all and the germ is nothing.

On the other hand, it is simplistic to state that natural immunity explains the fact that some individuals contract the disease and most do not, even when exposed to the same infectious agents.

I will not discuss the benefits that the Pasteurian germ theory of disease has given to humanity. Because it is applicable only on a small scale, the widespread abuse of the theory has led to an aggressive form of therapeutics that goes far beyond its benefits. A few years ago, an American physician thought he had isolated a bacillus epilepticus in the intestine of an epileptic patient. In keeping with his training concerning the nature of disease, he could not understand that epilepsy is not an infectious disease but a psychological and nervous reaction strictly related to the patient's personality or to a neurological lesion.

I have seen an antialpha and epsilon vaccine prescribed for sinusitis in a young girl who had already exhausted the whole store of vaccines and antibiotics. This same concept is still applied today with focal infections, according to which tonsils, teeth, appendixes, gallbladders and even pieces of intestines are mutilated. It is astonishing to observe the general agreement in the medical world regarding these practices, together with the inability to recognise that the focal infection is not a cause but a consequence of the disease, and that the patient's improvement is not due to the suppression of a focal infection but to the effectiveness of the law of cure.

However, in spite of the tremendous use of antibiotics, cortico-steroids and psychopharmaceuticals, the clinical approach of treating the patient's personal aspect – and not the disease as an abstract entity divorced from the person – has made some advances.

Hahnemann has not been the only one to advocate the study of the whole disease in the light of the patient's whole symptom picture and life history. Many others have done so, from Galen himself, the creator of analytical medicine, to Claude Bernard, the champion of experimental medicine, who stated: 'Organic physiology can be expressed in physical and chemical terms, but the total ordering of the organism as a whole is unquestionably vital and obeys laws that go beyond those of physiology and the organs.'

Behind the symptoms, before organic expression, the true disease runs its course. This is the disease *per se*, the dynamic root of the morbid disposition, that vital substratum which, lacking physical symptoms, expresses itself through the individual's way of life and which is unconsciously determined by the strength or courage with which that person faces their process of adaptation to life.

The supposed dichotomy between the physiological and the

psychical is a thing of the past. Psychiatry, psychology and psycho-analysis tend to confirm the evolutionist idea that the psychic behaviour of nervous cells or neurons does not differ, in its nature, from the biological behaviour of any other specialised cell in the organism. All cells in the organism react together to the stimulus that satisfies the whole person's morbid susceptibility, such that we may say that every-thing biological is psychic and everything psychic is biological.

The Russian physiologist I. P. Pavlov (1849–1936) discovered the conditioned reflex, and explained the reflection of the environment on the mind and the laws that rule over integrated nervous action at the biological, physiological and psychological levels. He wrote:

> As an empiric psychologist, I have always been and am now an observer of myself and of others to the degree that this is prag-matically possible.
>
> The old adage *nosce te ipsum* – know thyself – is to inquire into others. I am deliberately against any theory which aims to encompass all the phenomena that make up our subjectivity. But I cannot give up the analysis of our subjectivity, nor the attempt to understand it in certain distinct points, predominantly through my own self.

It is important to quote this from a man whom I consider to be the most brilliant representative of pure scientific thought and who, through analysis and induction, explained animal and human behaviour based on the events of the biosocial environment in which they develop. Pavlov understood the need for the physician's subjective self-control in order to empathise with the patient's subjectivity. I consider Pavlov's image of *homo reflexologicus* as one of the most respectable and fruit-ful scientific inquiries into human subjectivity and the nature of disease.

Other great researchers who have sought the determining factor of disease in the personality are Sheldon, Jung and Kretschmer. Kretschmer (1888–1964), for example, assigned a certain number of diseases to specific categories of the personality. He found that short, thickset individuals with a broad trunk and shoulders had a tendency to develop vascular and manic-depressive conditions. In tall, thin, asthenic individuals, he noticed a predisposition to schizoid states and tuberculosis. These Kretschmerian categories – connecting the individual's psyche and body structure with the tendency to certain diseases – have been amply verified in clinical practice and have been pragmatically surpassed only by homoeopathy's constitutional bio-types such as Calcarea Carbonica, Lycopodium, Natrum Muriaticum, Phosphorus and others.

Undoubtedly, the positivist tradition in scientific research which prevails today and which is exemplified by Claude Bernard has estranged medicine from the ancient philosophical art that was practised in Aesculapius's healing temples. At the dawn of religion and philosophy, Hippocrates taught that the human personality was structured according to the spiritual and social milieu in which the individual lived. It was here that the law of similars was stated for the first time, evidently emerging from a holistic position concerning disease in the human being, and therefore a correct intuitive perspective of the principle of unity, ruling the real dynamic cause of the individual's physical and psychological behaviour.

Hahnemann took up the thread of this research and identified the dynamic substratum or morbid disposition, inductively proposing his theory of the miasms and psora as the true, dynamic underlying disease. With the scientific knowledge of his time, he described disease as a state which today we would call allergy, or the hyperexcitability produced by the immune system when faced with suppressions of outward releases of catabolic products derived from a disturbed vital energy.

Psora is produced when the *vis medicatrix*, or law of spontaneous cure, has been transgressed due to the old suppression of outward releases which Hahnemann described as skin eruptions, but he evidently was referring to the allergic irritability that has remained in the human being due to the primary suppression of instincts. Sudden, acute or convulsive reactions that surface as episodic eruptions are centrifugal releases of morbid energy, due to an abnormal stimulation of the organism.

Psora, syphilis and sycosis are vibratory derangements of vital energy. In psora, Hahnemann's basic miasm, a stimulus to the normal physical and mental homoeostatic function results in instability and anxiety. In syphilis, there is a decrease in the reactive function which we may call 'anergy', characterised by mental and physiological inhibition, retardation, destruction and suicide. In sycosis, there is a 'dysenergy' which leads to a hypertrophied ego and the disorderly proliferation of tissues that culminates in cancer.

Hahnemann's miasms are derangements of the vital force that express themselves as ways of life, primordial states of biological consciousness which leave their imprint on the organism's physiology, anatomy and morphology. Psora's fundamental sign is that basic, primary suppression which we human beings have brought about by attempting to differentiate ourselves as individuals or separate entities, thus losing our sense of cosmic interconnectedness with the undifferentiated vital current. This original sin of humankind has led to a state of anxiety, entailing our feeling of insecurity, the innermost core of neurosis.

The entire problem of disease lies in the basic feeling of insecurity, inferiority or lack of ability, which arises from that profound sense of loneliness which afflicts human beings from the moment they separate from their mothers at birth with the first cry of anguish. Starting our school days, facing puberty, adulthood, menopause, old age and any other critical moments in our process of growth, always generates a fear of the unknown. Physical ailments are ways in which human beings physically express their vital dilemma: to assert the personality, based on the instinct for power, domination and force – and at the same time to redeem oneself from the guilt that this produces by returning to an undifferentiated life in the maternal womb or by searching for the realisation of the transcendent self in a higher, spiritual plane of existence.

This dilemma of insecurity and guilt is symbolically represented by the myth of Prometheus who, because he wished to steal the fire from Zeus, was condemned to have an eagle eat his liver. The story of Prometheus is symbolically realised in Lycopodium, whose personality wavers between insecurity and the defence mechanism of pride, together with the malfunctioning of the liver, thereby assuaging the guilt feelings produced by the lust for power that compensates the ego's profound feeling of inferiority, which virtually eats the liver away.

In every human being, this constitutional feeling of insecurity or diminished worth has a psoric origin. This vital disharmony is the root of the existential anguish experienced by individuals in the face of the social suppression of their instincts. However, what really determines this basic feeling of insecurity is the syphilitic imprint on the vital energy (and consequently on the budding personality, with its weakened, hypofunctional character) that entails a hereditary, organic deterioration, thus moulding the tubercular symptom picture. All children are tubercular: they are born with diminished organic functions, which are psora together with syphilis – the so-called structural pseudo-psora – whose psychological trait is that same basic feeling of insecurity or inferiority.

Classical theories regarding diathesis in children such as exudative, angioneurotic, lymphatic, thymolymphatic and arthritic conditions, as well as bradytrophy, spasmophilia and excitability of the vagus nerve, refer to this very state of pathological predisposition – a deficiency of the vital force that characterises the syphilitic disposition that affects every child, as a natural way of life and not as an infectious state.

Born with a tubercular disposition of deficiency, the child develops a personality that is entirely compensatory. From earliest consciousness the child tries to make up for his organic and physiological deficiency by overasserting the ego's individuality, leading on the biological level to a hyperkinesis of the cells and eventually to cancer.

Pathologists know that underlying cancer we will always find the tubercular miasm or tuberculosis. Underlying the immature adult's hypertrophied, self-centred personality which has an insatiable thirst for affection and the gratification of power and ambition, there is a latent feeling of inferiority and insufficiency, characteristic of the childhood stage.

Both the tubercular and cancerous states, basic diathesis of all pathology, are syphilis and sycosis, syndromes which, when combined with the so-called psoric condition, determine a destructive or proliferative tendency of the cells. The physician must have access to that deep biological substratum from where the instinctive will to live emerges, and which moulds the individual's character or social personality and determines the organic pathology.

In terms of knowing what is to be cured in each patient, what is important for the homoeopath is not the disease as such nor the classification of disease, but the chronological sequence of diseases in a patient's clinical history. Therefore, the tendency to fall ill involves several other factors of an emotional and mental nature which cannot be explained in the physiological and pathological language of experimental medicine.

These psychic factors underlying clinical symptomatology are related to the development of the personality, and obey laws and a purposive sense that do not belong to the physical and chemical realms but go beyond the boundaries of scientific medicine. Thus medicine is rendered into the philosophical art of understanding, in a broad holistic way, the existential drama of each individual patient.

An essential factor in human disease, then, is the basic feeling of insecurity – the sensation of being alone and defenceless when faced with life's adverse circumstances. The fear generated by this sensation of loneliness causes the human being to react aggressively, in order to defend and assert his threatened individuality, thus stimulating the instinct for self-preservation. This increased self-consciousness imprisons the person in the narrow confines of egoism and buries him in the misery and anxiety of someone who feels increasingly lonely and in constant danger. The greater the concern for oneself, the more dangerous the threats of the world to one's personal integrity are imagined to be. The more we hide behind the defensive shield of our own limitations, the more diseased we become, and therefore all the more certainly oriented towards self-destruction.

This obsessive concern for oneself comes from the fear, generated by parental and moral censorship, of satisfying the instinct for self-assertion and defence in a competitive relationship with others, beginning with the desired triumph over the personality of the male parent. In its syphilitic expression, the destructive tendency called the death instinct is a lust for power that compels the individual to waver between a permanent feeling of guilt about their dynamic personality, their erotic and aggressive impulses, and the social conventions of the community, which forbid instinctive expansion. The result of this conflict is the reactive or social personality, that overlays the instinctive or dynamic personality. Each individual, so to speak, wears a protective armour with which they attempt to reconcile their instincts with social requirements by appearing to be meek and submissive. However, due to the emotional tension of the forced repression of these instincts, the individual is headed towards organic disease.

The balance between the instinctive and social strata of the personality makes the individual find himself in an apparent state of health that is related to a good adjustment to the social system. The homoeopathic remedy, always directed towards the correction of that miasmatically altered pathogenic dynamism of the instincts, impulses, desires or ambitions, can bring about a less compulsive requirement that will allow for adjustment. But even this does not achieve that perfect balance which we call health.

In the critical moments of an individual's existence, he may again feel insecure, alone, abandoned and ill, and overcome with the lust for power, that will never solve his underlying problem of existential anguish.

When the constitutional simillimum matches the resentments, hates, fears and anguishes derived from the conflicts between the dynamic personality and the social personality, it is capable of rectifying the *vis medicatrix* and establishing an adaptive equilibrium which nevertheless, as we have said before, is not true health. Emotional tensions will give way, organic and functional ailments which are their consequence will disappear and the reversible pathological structures will return to normal. However, the individual must continue the process of growth, which always implies a simultaneous state of disease and healing – an unstable balance between the latent, psoric, existential anguish due to the repression of instincts and the gratifications that the social personality will allow.

Only when we realise that our psychological and biological maturity does not consist of defending our separate individuality, preserving our self-centredness or solving our existential insecurity by accumulating material goods and obtaining power, but in developing a sense of community that will allow us to be rid of our self-consciousness, we are able to fulfil our highest purpose of existence. As Hahnemann maintained, this is possible once the will has been rectified by the simillimum.

To the degree that we can discover our innermost self and develop the awareness of that stratum of our personality where life palpitates at its most basic and undifferentiated level, where the voice of the absolute incites us to lose our individuality in order to gain universal consciousness (in losing our soul we shall gain it), will we attain true health. The development of that level of consciousness is a psychiatric reality that should not be relegated only to art or religion, but can be especially entrusted to the homoeopathic physician. In understanding the patient's whole life context, with self-knowledge and empathy, and with the correct remedy, the homoeopath can lead the patient to the realisation of their personal destiny.

Chapter 9

What to Cure in Each Patient
(1958)

To tackle the psychosomatic problem in homoeopathy is to bring basic Hahnemannian principles to the fore. Because polypharmacy adheres to a localised and organic concept of disease, it lacks these Hahnemannian principles. When one has gained a proper insight regarding what to cure in each patient, it is essential to prescribe a single remedy for each case in order to stimulate the natural law of cure.

Every remedy in the materia medica has its own unique personality: that is, a synthesis of a human being's complete biological reaction as it arises from the deepest levels of his whole system, where mental and physiological impulses blend in a primary core of the will.

From the earliest days of medicine, Hippocrates pointed out that underlying each patient is a humoral dyscrasia that conditions his unique pathology, with innumerable individual variations. According to Hahnemann, what must be cured is not the diseased organ nor the localised lesion, but the morbid dynamics that conditions the terrain and determines the structure of the individual personality.

Clinical research that stops at the weakened or damaged organ, that is limited to examining the physical and pathological symptom picture by any method, leads at best to a partial diagnosis of a specific moment in the patient's clinical history – as, for example, in an acute disease or in whatever current diseased state the patient suffers. However, it will fail to grasp the constitutional morbid dynamic that encapsulates the patient's whole life history and can be given only by that individual's characteristic totality.

Intellectually, the modern physician knows that they must help the patient more than the disease; they know that there is no such thing as a Cartesian split between a soul and a body, but only a vital dynamism that expresses itself simultaneously as psyche and organism. A patient does not have a stomach ulcer or asthma as a consequence of moral or nervous derangements, but a vital derangement which expresses itself organically as a physical disturbance and psychologically as a moral conflict. If the physician wishes to understand the morbid constitutional dynamism that produces both levels of expression, he must gain a profound knowledge of both these apparently separate but correlated processes, which are really expressions of the same phenomenon. As Hahnemann maintained, mental diseases are bodily diseases whose expressions are obscured by mental symptoms.

Even though current psychosomatic thought adheres to the body-mind dichotomy, it knows perfectly well that the human being thinks and feels with his whole biology, so to speak, and that psychological symptoms are also biological expressions.

A scrutiny of the unconscious mechanisms that determine the patient's vital attitude and behaviour will reveal how closely psychological and physiological phenomena correspond to one another, thus discrediting the separation of psychology and organic medicine. As Hippocrates' aphorism claims, *Consensus unus, conspiratio una* – the body is a single organ, and life is a single function. A purely analytic and organic medicine has led people to believe that a disease is cured by treating or surgically removing the diseased organ.

If this so-called medicine for the body has had any effectiveness, it is due to the partial suppression of the physiopathological expressions of the disease. But instead of spontaneously obeying the centrifugal law of cure, the morbid energy regresses, aggravating disease at its deepest plane, producing the increase in mental disease and malignant tissues that is now so prevalent.

In order to truly understand the current disease, the physician must never – absolutely never – overlook the patient's whole life history: his occupation, life circumstances, moral vicissitudes and personality.

What must be cured in a patient is not the current disease but the profound, personal, inner condition which has brought about that particular pathological expression. Every day, surgery is performed on a multitude of stomach, liver and intestinal cases – surgery that could have been avoided if these patients' moral circumstances and vital attitudes had been fully understood. The human being is not an organism, but has an organism which serves the ends of a personal and vital formula, established by the interaction of biological impulses and guided by moral conscience. The homoeopath must be sensitive to the essential, general nature of the disease. There is no cure unless harmony has been restored in the whole individual and all symptoms have been eradicated.

In Paragraph 11 of the *Organon*, Hahnemann says: '… it is only the vital principle, deranged to such an abnormal state, that can furnish the organism with its disagreeable sensations, and incline it to the irregular processes which we call disease ...'

First, as always happens during the invasive period of acute disease, the inner planes are altered. Later on, the organic and superficial lesions appear. Therefore, the disease must be addressed at its initial internal root before the subsequent exterior disturbance becomes apparent. When this centrifugal path from the centre of the organism to the periphery is directed by the appropriate remedy, the patient's symptoms will disappear and a cure is brought about.

The natural consequence of applying a therapeutic system based on a true understanding of the patient's profound dynamic disturbance is to activate Hippocrates' *vis medicatrix naturae* or Hering's law of cure. From here emerge the impulses and drives of a miasmatically deranged instinctive will – in other words, the morbid substratum which must be cured in each patient. As long as the homoeopath fails to perceive that morbid substratum or fails to apply the series of remedies that match its dynamic action, he cannot expect to stimulate the law of cure. If this is achieved, the patient's cure is a realistic goal.

Characteristic totality does not consist of a mere aggregate of all the symptoms that the patient manifests; nor is it an arrangement that more or less matches the individualisation of all the patient's signs and symptoms. What the patient expresses spontaneously, as well as his localised symptoms, do not constitute the elements that must especially be taken into account. The patient must be interpreted and translated into the symptoms of the materia medica and the repertory. The homoeopath does not look for symptoms in the usual sense, in order to add up the patient's characteristic totality, but seeks the modalities, conditions or attitudes which may improve, aggravate or even provoke symptoms for the patient – in other words, to detect the particular way in which each individual conditions and bears their illness.

It is precisely these modalities of the particular symptoms, those strange and peculiar sensations described by Hahnemann, as well as the patient's mood, that make up the unique dynamic entity which has determined the current pathological process.

The science and art of homoeopathic symptomatology consists of understanding the causes, conditions, circumstances and evolution of symptoms that culminate in the lesion. The symptom picture or syndrome picture that corresponds to the diagnosis of the current disease can never be the characteristic elements that fully identify the patient's individuality. Likewise, a single modality, an odd sensation or even a mental symptom cannot by itself characterise a patient. What is truly characteristic is a total integration of clinical data, segregated from the common syndrome of the disease, but also taking the disease's modalities which qualify it into account. It is mistaken to consider a single symptom as decisive in the characterisation of a symptom picture. The much-abused keynote symptom, for example, is only an indicator that helps to identify and qualify a symptom picture. Because its only purpose is to help to individualise a case, it has no clinical value in itself, but only as part of a whole.

It is mistaken to assign an absolute value to a symptom just because it is mental or general according to Kent's hierarchy, or because the symptom strikes us as peculiar because it lacks a physiological explanation. To proceed in such a fashion reveals a deficient understanding of homoeopathy.

Strange and peculiar symptoms must be understood in terms of an individual's psychological evolution.

How a symptom will rank will depend on its function in a totality that gives personal character to a morbid process.

The relationship of the totality to the disease is the same as the relationship of the human self to the organism. One patient may have a common symptom that is part of a characteristic totality of another patient. No symptom or modality has an isolated value, but only in relation to a patient's whole life history. What is really characteristic is the patient's 'personal quotient', so to speak – their unique, peculiar type of dynamic reaction, and this is what must be cured.

Sound homoeopathy may require that a patient with an inflamed gallbladder, for example, be treated with a remedy that has nothing at all to do with inflamed gallbladders, but instead corresponds to the miasmatic dynamism which tends to produce destructive or proliferative inflammatory lesions in that patient.

The essential goal of homoeopathy is to identify the patient's morbid substratum – the miasmatic dynamism which determined the patient's character before the physiopathological lesion. Here lie the elements which make it possible for the homoeopath to know what must be subjected to the law of cure in each patient.

Paragraph 3 of the Organon

The objection has been raised that homoeopathy is based on localised or pathological symptoms and that it acknowledges only the diagnosis of the patient, and in so doing denies the need for physiopathological diagnosis. For those who do not understand homoeopathy, it is not

surprising that we appear unscientific when, without additional explanation, we state that the homoeopath's clinical practice is to diagnose
without reference to the pathological lesion. Along with this objection
come the remarks of those who accuse homoeopaths for not examining
their patients at all – in short, that by neglecting scientific scrutiny they
disregard the physiopathological process.

A few basic notions can bear repetition here. According to Hippocrates, the patient's diseased organ cannot be divorced from the whole
patient in space and time. Supported by inductive reasoning, his synthetic approach to medicine was an active forerunner of today's studies
of the constitutional terrain, susceptibility, humoural dyscrasias, neu-
rology and endocrinology, homoeopathy, reactions to stress and current
psychosomatic thought. In contrast, the analytical school of medicine
still seeks the *specie morbosa* that must be suppressed, considering the
patient as a passive entity. Modern medicine has understood that both
schools must settle their differences. To quote Claude Bernard's famous
dictum: the last element of the morbid phenomenon is physical, its
ordering is vital.

Homoeopathy is both analytic and synthetic. Not only does a complete clinical history enable the physician to study the patient's current
and past symptoms, it also helps to rank the characteristic symptoms
that individualise the patient above the common symptoms of the
disease. The patient's total dynamic reaction makes up his 'personal
quotient', translated as a useful syndrome for therapeutics. This does
not underestimate the diagnosis of the disease and the pathological
lesion. Far from the dogmatic spirit so often attributed to it,
homoeopathy turns to all branches of medicine in order to establish a
pathological, neurological and psychological diagnosis, thus distinguishing between the common symptoms of the disease and the
characteristic symptoms of the patient which have no pragmatic value
for conventional medicine but which make up homoeopathy's exclusive
symptomatological domain.

In keeping with the main goal of curing, above and beyond Galenic
medicine's deductive classification based on physiopathological syndromes, homoeopathy offers a new inductive classification based on the
similarity between natural syndromes and the syndromes which are the
result of remedy provings on healthy human beings. This synthetic
approach mirrors the ancient Hippocratic concept of dyscrasia or
humoral imbalance.

Pathogenesis, or the symptom picture that a drug produces in a
remedy proving, is homoeopathic classification. As Hippocrates stated,

that which produces the urethral spasm which really does not exist, cures the urethral spasm which really does exist. Twenty-four centuries later, we may say, with Hahnemann, that the case that Hippocrates cured with black hellebore was not called acute gastroenteritis, but the disease Helleborus, because this is the remedy that cures a special type of patient with violent gastroenteritis.

In Renaissance times, Paracelsus said that because there are as many diseases as diseased people, what the patient suffers as a vital unit cannot have the name of a disease, but the name of the chemical substance that produces similar effects.

The way in which homoeopathic remedies are prepared frees their molecular energy. Dynamised in this way and taken in minimum doses, they are capable of producing the modalities that are specifically human, allowing the diagnosis of each particular reactive syndrome. Likewise, toxicology offers us symptom pictures that reflect the experimental pathogenesis. For example, arsenic destroys tissues, produces gangrene, ulcerations and a septic state in the blood; at infinitesimal doses, it is a remedy which matches, and therefore addresses, a syndrome denoting that very same destructive tendency in a patient.

Opium is a narcotic that causes passive cephalic congestion, deep stupor, facies vultuosa, bloodshot and half-open eyes, stertorous breathing and hot, profuse perspiration; at infinitesimal doses it is the first remedy that comes to the homoeopath's mind when faced with an apopleptic symptom picture.

The poison of the snake *Lachesis trigonocephalus*, which recently gained notoriety in the treatment of malignant tumours, unleashes secondary diencephalic bulbar reactions with spasmodic, vasomotor and haemotoxic symptoms. This is a menopausal picture with hypomanic excitement, suffocation, hot flushes, bleeding and bruising.

Belladonna causes poisoning with dryness of the throat and mouth, dilated pupils, active congestion of the face, fast heartbeat, dry, hot skin, vertigo, hallucinatory delirium, eruptions and convulsions. This syndrome has its analogy in scarlet fever.

Gelsemium causes drooping of the eyelids and lower jaw, muscular relaxation, weakness, morbid dilation of the pupil, rapid but feeble pulse with low blood pressure; in a homoeopathic dose, it is one of the main remedies for debilitating nervous influenza.

All the remedies that make up the homoeopathic materia medica can be described in this way – that is, each with its own complete image of the general and localised psychological symptoms that confer a definite personality to each remedy.

This is the functional dynamic aspect that precedes and accompanies the pathological disease. It is the only possible and useful diagnosis which enables the physician effectively to cure the patient of, say, a stomach ulcer, gall or kidney stones, cysts, growths, eczema, or other ailments.

The patient will not be cured by the surgical removal of ulcers, stones, cysts and growths, nor by the suppression of skin eruptions. Measures such as these will only suppress the results of the dynamic disturbance that existed before the lesion appeared and which previously had the vague, diffuse characteristics of a general disease which at that time was not diagnosable. This disturbance subsists in latent form until it subsequently finds a new localisation that leads to pathological diagnosis.

Only when the totality of symptoms is eradicated can Hahnemann's essential goal of medicine be attained. This totality of symptoms is not only made up of the localised and general expressions of the organic disease, but also by the symptoms that reveal the patient's constitutional morbid background – those hidden symptoms which correspond to the individual's dynamic predisposing affection.

Backed up by the indisputable success of experiments performed on animals, current medicine focuses all its attention on analytic research into morbid processes. It seeks to know each and every physiopathological mechanism, taken logically as isolated circuits, but often fails to refer this research to the totality of the human organism and to consider that each one of its parts has a profound influence on the neurological, endocrine and hepatic balance that regulates the life of the whole.

The fact is often overlooked that morbid processes are not partial static imbalances, as if they were morbid species grafted on to the individual, but parts of a dynamic unit with a past and a future, interpenetrated by the cosmos and participating in the universal motion of sympathy that reigns over the whole of creation.

Cartesian rationalism has exerted too much influence on the scientifically oriented physician. Capable of exhaustive scientific scrutiny, the modern physician nevertheless lacks the spirit of synthesis that would permit him to integrate analytic discoveries into the living wholeness of the human being. Nature is unity in infinite diversity, perpetual movement and change, life and death, action and reaction, love and hate, reason and emotion, health and disease.

Health, disease and healing are the same vital process of a perpetual effort to maintain the dynamic equilibrium of the whole organism.

Medicine has become a portentous system that has enriched science with a large body of observations. However, it has mistakenly believed that gathering analytic elements together is an end in itself. The physician must return to ancient Hippocratic thought, which fosters a holistic approach regarding all morbid processes, the prevalence of constitutional factors and the purposes or final causes in all vital reactions.

In his time, Hahnemann produced a renaissance of these ancient Hippocratic principles which today seek new expression. Hahnemannian homoeopathy is not reduced to the use of remedies at infinitesimal doses, but is grounded in the deep respect for the uniqueness of each individual's natural, dynamic, total reaction. For the first time in the history of medicine, Hahnemann found a solution to the problem first perceived by Hippocrates, maintaining that, because it is impossible to know the causal antecedents of diseases, we should treat the effects of the disease which are studied in the patient with the effects of known remedies. It is only through symptoms, and symptoms alone, that disease makes itself known. By removing the effects, we remove the disease which is the cause of those effects.

Hahnemann deeply respected the *vis medicatrix naturae*. In the *Organon* he requires that the patient's hygiene, nutrition and occupation be assessed, as well as their intellectual, moral and environmental circumstances, in order to discover the underlying cause of disease – the chronic miasm, the profound dynamic derangement which has made the patient ill.

As he stated, supported by his numerous drug provings, the diseased human being creates a pathogenic equilibrium with the chronic disease, thus needing the very remedy that will trigger an analogous reaction. In this way, the *vis medicatrix* vitalises its energy.

And finally, well aware of his mission, Hahnemann inveighed against an empiric therapeutic system that subordinates the remedy to a partial and pathological diagnosis and suppresses reactive symptoms that denote the organism's effort to restore its balance – all in the name of cure. In his later years, he lamented not having more energy to cry out to the medical and scientific world the damage done to humanity with a toxic and suppressive therapeutic system that takes only the final products of pathology into account.

As far as scientific progress goes, today's exaggerated increase in analytic research is highly commendable. However, it is secondary to the fulfilment of the physician's essential mission to cure. And to cure a human being is to understand the essence of the human condition.

Consider Paragraph 9 of the *Organon*:

> In the healthy condition of man, the spiritual vital force (autocracy), the dynamis that animates the material body (organism), rules with unbounded sway, and retains all the parts of the organism in admirable, harmonious, vital operation, as regards both sensations and functions, so that our indwelling, reason-gifted mind can freely employ this living, healthy instrument for the higher purposes of our existence.

To cure is to help a fellow human being harmoniously to integrate their personality in a unit of thought and will, purpose and action, which will in turn lead to psychological maturity – that is, to the development of their spiritual potential for freedom and transcendence.

These are the lofty aims of human existence established by Hahnemann. The pathology of the personality is as important as cellular pathology. If a person is a physician, it is not because they are merely a practitioner of a technique or a scrutinising diagnostician, but because within them there lives the true meaning of medicine.

Chapter 10

Homoeopathic Diagnosis
(1959)

Because of the special value of subjective symptoms in building up the symptom picture, understanding the individual as a person is essential. In practice, a superficial case-taking is not enough to bring out these symptoms, generally of a psychic nature. This is the greatest difficulty in taking the case.

Sound clinical practice in homoeopathy is attained when the homoeopath is able to discern the patient's true symptoms. In so doing, the physician will be certain of the prescription and will rationally follow the development of each case, observing, for example, how these dynamic symptoms move according to the patient's tubercular or sycotic background, and not according to the metastatic and alternating mobilisation of pathological symptoms.

It is in this dynamic substratum of pathogenic activity that the more defined symptomatology occurs. It is here that the homoeopath must base their diagnosis, free from prejudices that could hinder a proper examination of the patient's personality.

There is no method so certain and effective as scrutinising the patient's symptoms by delving deeply into his subjectivity. No technological procedure can replace the imponderable value of human contact between physician and patient in the face of disease. That is why homoeopathic symptomatology must be adapted to the fullest knowledge of the personality. Patients tend to have their own notions regarding their symptoms. However, these notions are linked to unconscious feelings and motivations which the physician must discover through the history. Isolated symptoms have no value unless they refer to this deep, dynamic context.

A true homoeopathic interview is one in which the physician directs the patient's attention to himself, not as a clinical case but as a person. The remedy that cures a patient with neuralgic symptoms is the same remedy that corresponds not so much to the modalities of pain as to the patient's general characteristics, linked to the chronic process that gave rise to those symptoms. Every localised process must be examined in order to perceive the clinical elements of continuity that establish the unity of the living being who suffers a localised illness. Here lies the difference between those who believe that all symptoms must be addressed by the remedy and those who maintain that, because the mere sum of symptoms has no consistency, there must necessarily be a characteristic pattern that predominates.

Homoeopathy is the only therapeutic system based on direct experimentation on human beings. If it is reduced to matching current symptoms with remedies, it will not only err, but will also not go beyond being a mere empiric application of those remedies.

It is not enough to have a symptomatic view of the remedies and master their keynotes, characteristics and modalities. It is essential to apply oneself to understanding the remedy's dynamic action and the patient's whole personality. One female patient came to my office with functional stomach disorders, aggravated by sweets. She also felt aversion, and even admitted feeling hate, towards her mother, from whom she had distanced herself due to bitter disputes concerning her father's inheritance. Ignatia has hate, anger with silent grief, and a marked aggravation by sweets, a symbolic representation of maternal nourishment, thus corresponding to the symptom picture of this case.

As the homoeopath builds up an image of the patient, he identifies and ranks the organic, psychological and determinative symptoms of the case. From this dynamic perspective, only subjective symptoms, sensory impressions, sensations and behavioural expressions can occur, which reveal the patient's character and personality and which are essential in the diagnosis. Nevertheless, these dynamic traits are difficult to grasp, especially for physicians who have had an organic-based training and who, due to their own personal inhibitions, may hesitate to inquire into the patient's intimate life and therefore who are reluctant to include psychological factors in their patients' case histories.

A thorough and patient case-taking is the most valuable aspect of clinical practice, especially when the physician addresses neuroses such as hysteria, obsessions and phobias caused by frictions with the environment. Accurate prescriptions are obtained when the homoeopath goes beyond organic prescribing to reassess the patient's concealed mental symptoms, which are missing from the current symptom picture. Only then may the true picture emerge.

One woman had a crisis of paroxysmal tachycardia with profuse perspiration. Her attacks lasted 10-12 hours, with a sensation of great physical restlessness and intense vertigo when lying down. A physical examination yielded nothing except oscillating hypertension, probably of emotional origin. However, the clinical history and her life story revealed an anxiety neurosis converted to paroxysmal tachycardia.

For the purposes of homoeopathic diagnosis, this patient did not have precise mental symptoms at that moment, but her life history revealed that before her ailments began she had an intense fear of dying when alone, which took the form of sudden suicidal thoughts.

Knowing the correlation between anxiety and tachycardia, the fear of death was not necessary at that moment, in order to know that this key symptom was nevertheless implicit and still very much in force in her life history, from which it was not difficult to diagnose Arsenicum. The woman was outwardly calm but had such a fear of death that, because she could not bear it any longer, she had sudden attacks of suicidal thoughts, aggravated when alone.

Another patient, a young mother of two children aged three and five, had a symptom picture of anxiety, depression, violent headaches, a sensation that she was going insane, fear of death and being alone, vertigo, transient fainting spells, very painful and scanty menses with amenorrhoea of one to two months, aversion to people, hot flushes in the face, shiverings and uncontrollable jealousy. Her husband was a sailor. On one of his trips the year before, he had sent her a letter telling her that he had gone to a dance. This news made her feel so betrayed by him that, ever since, she had been left with the obsessive thought of her husband's possible unfaithfulness and the sensation of going mad, and she tried to stay away from people so as not to show her state of confusion. She was a patient who was markedly stouter in the lower half of her body, with a preference for salty and cold foods, irregular thirst, chronic constipation, general lethargy at 10 to 11a.m. and a marked tendency towards hurriedness and agitation. Except for her endocrinological disorders and her emaciated face and neck, a clinical examination revealed nothing objective or organic.

In this case, jealousy was an apparently determinative symptom, as well as her sad, timid, self-conscious, passive demeanour, all of which would make one think of Pulsatilla. On the other hand, if I had based my repertorisation only on current symptoms and had considered her sensation of insanity and her fear that people would notice her confusion as outstanding symptoms, I could have equally thought of Calcarea Carbonica, Natrum Muriaticum, Phosphorus or Sepia. As in all cases, the challenge was to build up the symptom picture properly and identify the determinative symptoms. This patient expressed jealousy as a key to her situation. However, was jealousy what really troubled her? Perhaps a deeper, more personal understanding of this symptom was called for. Homoeopathic diagnosis must never be based only on what the patient says – usually the result of poor self-observation – but must cut across the secondary neurotic elaboration of their real experiences.

A more detailed enquiry revealed that this patient had been thin and irritable as a child, with a crossed right eye from age 5 to 16, when she was operated on; that she was timid and suffered from sudden and desperate attacks of weeping; that then, and even now, consolation improved her condition but that she did not want either of her parents to come near her, because her desperation worsened and she felt an impulse to harm them; that she had an obsessive fear of the death of one of her parents, not only for them, but especially because of what could happen to her; and that she still could not recover from the feeling of rage and shame that were brought on by her classmates' making fun of her cross-eyed condition.

Undoubtedly, the primary symptoms had gone through a reactive change that produced a current false symptom picture. She was no longer a passive patient who sought consolation with the painful need for affection of a Pulsatilla, but a patient with much resentment and a large burden of repressed hostility towards her parents, manifested by the violent rejection that she expressed towards them in the middle of her sudden bursts of weeping, the guilt she felt for what could happen to her if one of her parents died, and the crossed eye itself as an exponent sign, so to speak – in keeping with the law of *pars pro toto* – of the aggressive tension of her muscular system.

Her jealousy was due to a need to free the reactive hate towards her parents, actualised by a trivial incident that triggered the resentment imprinted upon her subconscious as a conditioned reflex. In this case, her jealousy had no prescriptive value, because it was really not jealousy, but hostility; thus her true personality was thrown into relief. Pulsatilla needs the protection and demonstrative affection of everyone in order to relieve her feelings of inferiority, passivity and low self-esteem. Pulsatilla is jealous of anyone who gives attention and affection to another and not to Pulsatilla exclusively. On the other hand, the jealousy of Lachesis conceals impulses of infidelity, projects exacerbated erotic feelings during menopause, attributes to her spouse instinctive pressures which cause her anxiety, and thus justifies and obtains through jealousy a relief for her tension.

This patient's life history allowed us to become acquainted with her real character which, as is often the case, was hidden behind a compensatory defence mechanism. I was thus able to identify her true constitutional simillimum.

Her picture was made up of the following symptoms: malicious; anger with silent grief; fear of insanity; fear of evil; fear that something will happen; aggravated by consolation; hurried; general lethargy between 10 and 11a.m.; desire for salty foods; obesity in the lower part of the body, and a crossed eye (corrected by surgery).

The repertorisation led to Natrum Muriaticum. Nevertheless, even before I had repertorised, her real character, revealed through the origin and evolution of her symptoms, made the image of Natrum Muriaticum come to mind with a clarity that could never have been obtained through the simple transcription of current symptoms.

Because, generally speaking, patients seek a diagnosis that they themselves have built up (and may even unconsciously seek to confuse the physician), we must not take them as they come, but how they really are. A patient may have a syndrome of fatigue, headaches, indigestion, spasms of the gall bladder, vomiting and other symptoms, with no organic lesion or alteration, but may nevertheless repeatedly and stubbornly deny that he is being negatively affected by a life situation. Such patients tend to seek physicians who will confirm their own views and even perform surgery on them. In homoeopathy, the clinical problem does not stop at the pathological diagnosis but at the knowledge of the diseased person. We must be prepared for the unwitting lack of frankness or lack of self-knowledge in a patient that would help the physician to gain a clear and faithful picture of that person's state. And it is precisely this which interests the homoeopath, even more so than blood pressure, electrocardiograms, blood counts, electrolyte balance or analysis of the intestinal flora. Such data are undoubtedly of great clinical importance as analytical elements, but their medical value is always subject to the patient's totality.

Another patient, a 44-year-old mother of three, complained of bad headaches, intense burning sensations in the stomach after meals, pain in the hypogastrium with a marked bearing-down sensation, worse before painful menses, heaviness of the limbs with varicose veins, and vertigo upon getting up. She had also had several fainting spells while kneeling in church. Her only organic symptom was a heavy discharge. According to her and her family, she harboured a great fear of disease, was very emotional and depressed with constant weeping, and, at the same time, a marked obsession with the tiniest details of her household, seeing to it that food, clothing, floors, artefacts and so on were impeccable. She reacted with anger at the least transgression against the hygiene and order she had imposed at home. She had the reputation in her family of being haughty, violent, intolerant, impulsive and discontented. During the interview, she burst into tears and wept inconsolably, offering as an explanation that she really felt out of place and a stranger in her own house, which she admitted to not liking.

With this first symptom picture, Sepia was apparently determined by: weeping in the consulting room, fainting while kneeling in church, fear of disease, irritable, intolerant, indifferent to affection, bearing-down sensation, acid indigestion, heavy discharge, heaviness of the limbs and weak ankles.

However, I was not convinced that I was face-to-face with a Sepia image. She did not have the indifference, apathy and aloofness which are the usual background for Sepia cases. Her deep sadness with painful weeping during the interview did not reveal an attitude of renunciation and lack of interest in life, but rather a rebellion against her impotence to deal with her family and household duties. Sepia, in contrast, indifferently ignores household duties.

Her life history revealed nothing pathological, but she did say that she had been an only child whose father had died of liver cancer three years previously. After marrying at the age of twenty-six she had continued to live with her parents. Her mother, still alive and well, had always been concerned about her husband, whose liver illness had been chronic. Having been especially devoted and very attached to him, my patient claimed emphatically that her father had been the person whom she had loved most dearly in her life.

Because her husband was present during the interview, I took this as a flagrant snub against him, verified by her general attitude of haughtiness and pride. She had described herself as a frank and direct person, as one who could not bear to see her house in disorder and who did not allow anyone to do things for her. She was afraid of falling ill and not being able to tend to her house properly. Adamantly against the idea of hiring help, she had refused to go on holidays in order not to leave her post for a single moment.

This patient was obsessively attached to her household, with an inclination towards domination and aggressiveness that concealed an anxiety rooted in a deep feeling of insecurity. She was also proud and haughty as a reaction to her feelings of inferiority after the death of her father, who had always been obedient to the influence of his only daughter. She lacked confidence in herself and in others, because nothing had been able to satisfy her deep longing for self-affirmation and success.

In addition to these feelings of inferiority, and the compensatory symptoms with which she protected herself from anxiety, her true picture was made up of the following determinative symptoms: haughty, dictatorial, conscientious, want of self-confidence, grief, suspicious; heartburn, pain in the hypogastrium before menses and heaviness of the limbs.

I omitted the symptoms of fainting spells in church and weeping in the consulting room because (according to the patient herself) they were directly related to her father's death. Every time she prayed for her father she felt so sad that she wanted to die. Her fear of disease was due to the impossibility of fulfilling her duties with the extreme conscientiousness she demanded of herself. Therefore, on the basis of her true characteristic syndrome rather than on a mere repertorisation, Lycopodium overrode Sepia.

A 58-year-old man came to my office with rheumatism, frequent colds, coryzas, inflammation of the paranasal cavities and bronchitis. He was very sensitive to cold, and caught colds even when he became chilled in a specific part of his body such as his head or feet. He also complained of periodic migraine headaches that affected the left side of his head above the eyeballs or in the occiput; slow digestion, with belching, flatulence and rumbling in the bowels; cramps in his calves; drowsiness during the day with insomnia at night, and a marked state of agitation, nervousness and great restlessness. He insisted vehemently that he felt a need to hurry and was anxious to start anything, especially at his job.

Taken at face value, the principal symptom that stood out in this symptom picture, due to the intensity with which it was expressed, was hurry, agitation, desire to do things quickly – which is characteristic of sycosis and which appeared as an excluding symptom in this patient. However, delving further into the man's life history, I came to the conclusion that he was very ambitious, and that all his life he had nurtured a commendable wish to secure a good financial position. However, he also had an insurmountable disposition towards dependency, which undermined his ability to undertake freelance work. This vital conflict led him to assume an attitude of competitive rivalry vis-à-vis his boss and other people. But because of his dependent character, he also had to repress the aggressiveness roused by his frustrated wish for success.

The result was an obsessive neurosis, expressed by the excessive zeal and meticulousness with which he carried out the duties assigned to him at the company where he worked. He admitted that the hurry and agitation, which he had stated was the prime motivation for consulting me, overcame him when he had to render an account to the company cashier and when turning in large sums of money. It was then that the fear of being caught doing something wrong, of not rendering an exact account and losing his boss's trust, would arise. By extension, every time his manager assigned him some task directly, this patient said the same hurry and agitation would 'grip' him because he felt his reputation for trustworthiness was completely at stake. This did not occur when he worked at home or when he performed tasks that did not involve his boss.

Clearly, his anxious and agitated manner was a compulsive reaction to his own aggressive impulses of disloyalty and hostility towards the person on whom he depended, thus thwarting his own ambition.

His situation was not really characterised by hurriedness, because it surfaced only when he felt the unconscious need to bury his fear of attacking his boss. The true determinative symptom was his obsessive conscientiousness.

His real symptom picture, then, was made up of the following: conscientious; want of self-confidence; very sensitive to cold; catches cold easily from getting chilled in one part of the body, head or feet; and migraine headaches on the left side from above the eyeballs to the occiput.

Silica was the simillimum in this case. Interestingly enough, my diagnosis was confirmed when Silica brought on an old and foul foot sweat which he had had before but had not spoken of in the first interview. His neurosis and general state also showed a marked improvement.

If, in my search for the correct remedy, I had stopped at what seemed to be the determinative symptom which surfaced in the first phase of the case-taking, that is, hurry and agitation, I would have easily excluded Silica, which has no agitation, and would have erred in my diagnosis.

Therefore, symptoms must never be transcribed without understanding their meaning and origin, as shown by the patient's whole personality, thereby allowing the physician to understand the latent content of the expressed symptoms and to assess their true value.

It is easy to see that I have abstained from referring to symptoms which are the result of a physical examination. In this man's case, there was nothing pathological of relevance to a diagnosis. Nevertheless, above and beyond any physical expression of the patient's illness, the physiopathological diagnosis always refers to the constitutional personality that is made up of the symptoms of dynamic derangement – the essential aspect of the disease. It is to that plane, the very background of pathology, that the physician must turn. The patient's characteristic syndrome rises spontaneously and clearly in the physician's mind, as an inductive result of the synthesis of the patient's whole life: inherited traits, pathological background, infections, intoxications, moral and physical traumas, environmental and current emotional circumstances.

Symptoms are physiological mechanisms and reactive expressions of a primary dynamic process, whose roots will be found, beyond any physical clinical reality, in the patient's hidden personality. That is why the physician must trace the physiopathogenic origin of each symptom. For it is there, in the hidden personality, that Hahnemann identified the primary derangement of the vital energy, with the destructive, deadly spirit of syphilis, the perversion of sycosis and the underlying anxiety of psora – the fundamental disease of humanity and the origin of all morbid and pathological processes.

By systematically scrutinising the characterological background of all expressions of disease, even of such gross pathological manifestations as advanced tissue damage – where often it may actually be necessary to apply localised and palliative therapy – homoeopathy satisfies a plea for humanisation in all medicine. Furthermore, it also confirms its own clinical practice – by directly contacting the patient's emotional stratum – in order to understand the true nature of hidden symptoms, reactive transformations or defence mechanisms of the patient. In this way, homoeopathy attains a level of certainty in the whole diagnosis, one which cannot be obtained by any technical procedure that aims to replace the physician's direct perception and understanding of the problem.

Chapter 11

Selecting the Homoeopathic Remedy
(1960)

To discern clearly the patient's unique characteristic syndrome, and to choose the first remedy, requires a detailed and intelligent analysis of the patient's whole life history. The patient's unique characteristic syndrome is made up of mental symptoms derived from a disturbance in the three main ways in which vital energy seeks expression: emotions, will and intelligence. In the first place, emotions determine our disposition towards love, cordiality, optimism, trust, wellbeing, joy, good humour, affability, generosity, inner peace – and, to a certain extent, the ability to assume that genuine inner freedom which pulsates in every human being as a persistent call to become as one with the whole of life, to live life at its fullest.

It is this call that underlies a patient's attitudes and emotional symptoms; these usually reveal a lack of love and eventually play a negative role in their growth and realisation as a human being. In the second place, our will unfolds its potential for creative service – self-confidence, decisiveness, industry, order, a love of what we do and a constant, dynamic mental and physical disposition to attain a true awareness of being, and with it the direct perception of what to do with our lives. For our circumstances depend on what we are, and therefore on the degree of responsibility and self-awareness that we have developed. Thirdly, the degree of intelligence we possess is related to our ability for comprehension, acumen and a profound intellectual and intuitive perspective of the unity of all life, which sooner or later we must discover in our own selves.

Emotions, will and intelligence, then, make up the psychic structure of the human being. Along with general reactive symptoms and modalities, the mental derangements derived from these three elements set the basic pattern for the patient's clinical history.

Although mental symptoms alone do not determine the diagnosis, they certainly do rule the whole picture, just as conspicuous mental or physical keynote symptoms help to open a case – so long, of course, as the general symptoms agree. What is important is to confirm the choice of remedy by understanding that the patient's emotional and physical clinical history is their unique way of responding to their personal psoric idiosyncrasy, that is to say, to their latent loneliness anxiety.

It is through symptoms, and symptoms alone, perceived directly and understood inductively and not by any deductive method, that we discover the 'minimum syndrome of maximum value'. This syndrome is made up of three, four or five characteristic, mental and general symptoms which dominate the picture and individualise our patient. It is on this syndrome that we must base both our therapeutic diagnosis as well as the remedial action that we expect from the remedy. Homoeopathic remedies do not act due to their gross chemical properties, but as dynamic factors which unlock vital energy. The reaction that the remedy provokes, which Hahnemann called an 'artificial disease', is what overrides the 'natural disease' on a purely energetic level, rectifying its vibratory dynamics and stimulating its own latent capacity for health or *vis medicatrix naturae*. In this way, the law of cure is set in motion.

And this is what really cures. It is the power of health – it is our life. What acts is the natural will, redirecting the vital force towards a positive, life-affirming dynamic, and away from a negative, self-destructive dynamic, as happens when the morbid process attacks the vital organs. In the healing process, a centrifugal dynamic reaction is generated, progressing from the centre to the periphery, from the vital organs to the excretory organs, and finally towards the fulfilment of the patient's true purpose in life, towards the highest ends of his existence. As Hahnemann maintains, this is a person's true identity in the development of their consciousness of being, that urgent call which is life's mental expression.

Not only does life exist, it exists in an intelligent way. Because the meaning of life is not distinct from life itself, life itself is its own meaning. The meaning of life and the dynamics of life are identical. When we are in harmony with the dynamics of life as a whole, which is always connected to our individual lives, we automatically discover, each and every one of us, the meaning of life and of our personal lives as well. And then, automatically, our attitudes are in accordance with that perspective. When things go wrong or people do not respond to us as we feel they should, it is because we are not centred or authentic enough in our perspectives nor are we in harmony with our own rhythm and the general rhythm of life.

These thoughts, derived from clinical experience, affirm the unity of both the cosmic and human expressions of life. The homoeopath would do well to integrate a life-affirming perspective in his or her own personal training, so as to develop that capacity for empathy so necessary for understanding the patient and building up the symptom picture. Because there are no precise rules yet which indicate the most suitable potency or dose, each homoeopath must make the best use of his own clinical skills and experience. To prescribe the necessary potency, the homoeopath must assess the patient's vitality, as well as any possible pathological obstructions of the excretory organs and structural changes in the vital organs. As a general rule, the greater the similarity of the remedy to the patient's mental characteristics, the higher should be the potency employed, so long as there is no irreversible organic disease or tissue damage which could obstruct the healing reaction. The initial potency could be 1c, 30c, 200c, 1M or 10M, according to the physician's understanding of the patient and his perception of the patient's degree of vitality.

The First Prescription

The first prescription, or the choice of the patient's simillimum, is a task that demands the utmost skill. Grounded in a vocation both scientific and spiritual, the homoeopath will be able to perceive the remedial action in each remedy necessary for the case and know what must be cured in each patient.

Having found this minimum syndrome of maximum value – those characteristic symptoms which identify the profound psychological and biological individuality of each case – the physician must then turn to the repertory. As long as the mental symptoms have been correctly determined and agree with the general modalities which characterise the patient, and not with the numerical totality of pathological symptoms and particular modalities, repertorisation will determine the choice of the simillimum with precision.

Once the constitutional remedy has been correctly prescribed, the patient's symptoms will almost certainly change. Generally speaking, the symptoms that already existed tend to be aggravated and new symptoms appear. Here the physician must use his expertise to decide whether the law of cure has been activated – that is, whether the disease has been redirected from the centre to the periphery, from the patient's inner being, mind and vital organs, towards the excretory organs, skin and mucous membranes.

Some reactions to homoeopathic remedies are violent, others are not. Homoeopathic aggravations differ according to how strong the patient's vitality and mentality are and how long a chronic process has been going on. Other important factors are the presence of structural changes in the patient's vital organs, the amount of repeated suppressive medication, and the nature of the current circumstances.

A homoeopathic aggravation means that the remedy has provoked a dynamic reaction that overruns the actual disease, and thus generates a so-called artificial disease. These aggravated symptoms enhance the patient's defences and redirect the morbid dynamics towards the excretory organs and the organism's surface. Aggravations are thus outward releases towards the periphery. Although there may be structural changes in the skin or mucous membranes, vital organs such as the liver, kidneys, heart and brain remain unharmed.

Hahnemann and Kent described several different responses to remedies:

- The patient recovers promptly with no aggravation. A similar remedy was chosen. However, it did not affect the patient's constitutional state.
- A rapid, brief and strong aggravation, followed by a prompt improvement of the patient.
- A long aggravation with a final and gradual improvement of the patient.
- A long aggravation with a final deterioration of the patient. In this case, there is irreversible structural pathology which prevents recovery.
- A total relief of symptoms without any special improvement in the patient. This is also due to irreversible structural changes in the brain, heart, lungs, liver or kidneys.
- Improvement comes first, aggravation follows. The symptoms return, but are changed. The remedy has been palliative and has not stirred up old symptoms, or the patient has committed a dietary or hygienic transgression, or has interfered with the cure in some other way.
- A relief of symptoms that is too brief. Structural changes in the tissues or organs or in the deepest constitutional mental syndrome, with pathological lesions in the hypothalamus as occurs in obsessive neurosis, for example, may hinder or altogether impede the remedial action of a well-prescribed drug.
- Current symptoms are aggravated and disappear, followed by the appearance of old symptoms. When old symptoms reappear and

disappear, no medication whatsoever must be prescribed. When old symptoms return and remain stationary, the same remedy may be repeated.

- New symptoms appear that the patient did not have before. (The physician must be very sure of this.) The prescription was not accurate, or even detrimental. Symptoms must disappear of their own accord. If symptoms persist after waiting for two or three months and the patient does not improve, in spite of taking the remedy in progressive doses, it will be necessary to review the case and, only then, to change the remedy.

- The patient produces a pathogenesis (a 'proving') of the remedy. These patients tend to be sensitive and are difficult (but not impossible) to help. We must bear in mind that provers who are clinically healthy – or at the very least who maintain an apparent equilibrium – are always benefited by participating in provings, (as was Hahnemann himself, who experimented with more than sixteen remedies).

- Symptoms take a wrong turn, travelling from the periphery to the centre. (Diseases must be cured from the centre to the periphery – from the vital centres such as heart, lungs, brain, medulla, towards the extremities, skin and mucous membranes.) Inevitably, when a physician prescribes for conditions such as skin eruptions, mucous membranes or colds, while ignoring the patient's constitutional miasmatic state, the patient will continue to be ill and may even deteriorate towards irreversible structural changes.

Travelling from the centre to the periphery, from the mind to the organs, from the vital organs to the excretory organs, the *vis medicatrix naturae* moulds a dynamic consciousness of the unity of life. Thus, from a biologically conditioned, self-centred, irresponsible, dependent and passive child, an individual develops into a responsible, independent adult, a spiritually free being who is giving and open to the fullness of life.

When patients make a positive change in their lifestyle, vital attitude and manner, when they shift their level of awareness towards responsibility and growth, we may be sure that they are on the road to true recovery. When improvement is not limited to eradicating symptoms, but consists of the wellbeing that comes from developing one's creative powers; when patients actively dedicate their energy to unfolding their physical, emotional, mental, spiritual and aesthetic abilities and fulfilling their vocation with an attitude of service, then they attain true growth, strengthened by consciousness of happiness, fulfilment and authenticity, thanks to that unceasing will to live, now freed from the negative factors which had obstructed it. An individual's purpose in life is fulfilled when they affirm themself as the instrument of their destiny and not simply as a product of circumstances. A person who gains self-awareness becomes a luminous point that radiates outwards, a creative actor of his existence. According to Hahnemann, this is what true growth, adulthood, freedom, happiness, health and the attainment of the highest ends of existence consist of.

If patients do not show positive changes in their vital attitude, feelings and behaviour in this direction, no matter what their stage of development, then they are not healing. The law of cure motivates the individual towards full maturity as a human being. It is from this perspective that the homoeopath must consider the centrifugal path which the patient's symptoms travel.

The Second Prescription

For the second prescription, clinical experience has established that, if we have been unable to identify the chronic or constitutional simillimum, then the acute disease must be considered a defective disease. This is because the acute disease is a sudden release of the miasmatic constitutional disposition. In this case, so long as the patient's resistance is not jeopardised, the remedy that matches the current symptoms must be prescribed. In all other cases, we must wait until the acute episode passes with no medication whatsoever. The *vis medicatrix naturae* must not be interfered with, even more so if the patient is already undergoing homoeopathic treatment for chronic disease, whether with us or a previous prescriber. We must wait until the effects of previous doses pass.

Whether an acute episode arises in the course of a homoeopathic treatment or whether it occurs spontaneously, the law of cure is always fulfilled as a reaction of the *vis medicatrix naturae*. However, because constitutional chronic diseases do not heal of their own accord, their acute crises do not suffice to bring about a true cure. On the other hand, acute episodes which arise in the course of miasmatic or constitutional treatment do bring about effective cures. They must therefore not be interfered with by prescribing medications of any kind. Once the correct remedy has been found, it must be administered in a single high dose or whatever dose is considered appropriate. The patient can be said to be moving in the right direction if his general condition, mental state, sleep and appearance improve, and if there are discharges through the intestines, mucous membranes and skin.

When the improvement has been rapid, the same symptoms may return or the symptom picture may change. If the same remedy is indicated, it must be administered in a solution and repeated every two or three hours, shaking it in order to raise the potency, in every dose or spoonful, until there is an improvement. As soon as there is an improvement, all medication must be stopped.

If, in spite of improvement, the remedy has been repeated and the patient reflects the remedy's proving symptoms, upon detecting this mistake the physician must wait until these symptoms disappear of their own accord.

Whether with conventional or homoeopathic drugs, if the patient has been heavily medicated with doses too often repeated, it is helpful to administer the remedy that matches the current symptom picture.

If a well-chosen remedy has been administered in the appropriate dose and improvement has begun, new symptoms may nevertheless appear which were not present on the first prescription. These new symptoms may well belong to the remedy itself. They may not necessarily be identical to those produced by the remedy, that is, to their pathogenesis, but analogous. In any case, they will disappear of their own accord.

If these new symptoms show a worsening of the patient, the symptom picture must be reviewed. In accordance with the rest of the symptom picture, the symptom which remains constant will determine the new diagnosis.

When treating both acute and chronic diseases, it is often necessary to confront situations, as I have already mentioned, in which the patient does not manifest characteristic symptoms which correspond to the totality. Hahnemann called these cases defective diseases, in which the modalities of the current symptom picture or the localised disease prevail, concealing the patient's constitutional symptomatology, as in the acute cases just mentioned.

The patient's current state may not necessarily be the symptom picture of an acute disease, but the result of physical injuries, emotional trauma or intoxication by drugs, this latter being all too frequent nowadays, whereby the patient's reactive sensitivity has been dulled or disturbed by medication with psychotropic drugs, corticosteroids, vitamins, antibiotics and even incorrectly prescribed homoeopathic remedies. In these cases it is impossible to discern the true symptoms of the chronic constitutional disease. The homoeopath must identify the remedy which corresponds to the current symptom picture, nevertheless keeping the mental symptoms and general modalities in mind. This similar remedy will often cause the constitutional symptoms, on which the curative simillimum may be based, to appear.

This careful attention to the identification of symptoms requires all the physician's skill and expertise – he or she must not try to speed up the outcome of the case nor add on more remedies to the list, but be wise enough to wait.

Once the law of cure has been activated, we must always respect the *vis medicatrix*'s immutable direction, from the centre to the periphery, from the higher part of the body to the lower part, from the vital organs to the less vital organs or excretory organs, and the reappearance of symptoms in reverse order.

The same principles apply to chronic cases.

The improvement brought about by the remedy may eventually persist for weeks or months.

When a remedy is repeated, a higher potency must be administered.

If the improvement has been of short duration, the second dose must be of a higher potency, administered in a solution and repeated for a long time until it produces its effects; often it must be repeated for several weeks until improvement is clearly visible. Also, several doses may be given in succession, with a slight increase in the potency of each one.

It is absolutely necessary to wait until the first dose no longer acts, or until its effects have ceased before prescribing the second dose.

If its basic rules and principles are faithfully observed, homoeopathy cannot fail. To observe and wait is the order of the day.

The questions most frequently asked by homoeopaths are the following:

1) How long must I wait?
2) Is the remedy still 'acting'? In other words, is the vital energy still affected by the remedy?
3) If old symptoms are returning, how long will it be necessary to wait before administering a remedy?
4) Is the disease acute or chronic?
5) Why is the second prescription more difficult than the first?
6) Why are many patients helped by the first visit to the physician but fail to benefit from subsequent visits?

Good prescribers are capable of answering in the following ways:

1) We have acted swiftly, but we have never waited long enough.
2) After the first dose we can expect the following conditions:
   (a) An aggravation of current symptoms with a general improvement of the patient.
   (b) An aggravation accompanied by a general decline in the patient. The case may be incurable and must be handled with extreme care, because these patients rarely recover completely.
   (c) An improvement of some symptoms. This improvement is questionable and may imply incurability if the patient does not improve generally, or change their vital attitude and feel the return of the flexibility of life. Unless the totality of symptoms are stirred and the patient feels free from the negative factors that hinder the development of their innate capacity for energy, intelligence and emotion, true healing will not occur.
3) If the first remedy has been imprudently repeated, it is unlikely that the true image of the disease will return. Thus, the image that does appear will not be trustworthy.
4) If the first prescription was correct, returning symptoms will call for the same remedy.
5) If the remedy was only similar to an aggregate of superficial symptoms, the returning image reproduces the image of another remedy. If the physician should prescribe this remedy, the case will be twisted so badly that even a master prescriber would be incapable of rectifying it.
6) If the returning image is the same as the first image, the second dose must be administered in a higher potency, or else the same remedy may be prescribed at a plus potency.

Changing the Remedy

When the physician has waited long enough and symptoms return – even though they are not all the symptoms that comprise a patient's clinical history – the most recent returning symptom will guide the selection of the new remedy.

The symptoms that have reappeared will disappear shortly, although the most recent of them will not disappear. The physician must be sure that this symptom persists – the symptom picture established by this fixed, determinative symptom will enable the physician to choose the remedy.

As long as symptoms change, no remedy must be prescribed.

The acute symptoms of chronic miasms must be treated differently from acute diseases. If the colds, bronchitis, or asthma attacks that come with every weather variation are treated with acute remedies, this will only worsen the patient. The patient must be treated miasmatically – that is, with the deep-acting remedy that covers the constitutional disposition. The miasm that predisposes the patient to recurrent attacks must be considered.

In serious cases it is more frequent to err with the second prescription than with the first one, because of haste and not waiting long enough.

When the physician prescribes the first remedy, he must wait until the patient 'establishes' the symptom picture that follows the improvement after the first prescription. It is easy to fail here because of undue haste.

This also explains why many patients improve with the first prescription and then worsen, or else do not continue to improve. In these cases, the physician has not waited long enough. The patient improved at the beginning for a certain time and later has not responded to any subsequent remedies. Every change in the symptom picture, albeit with no new symptoms, has been accompanied by a new pre-scription.

If the patient has not improved, it is necessary to re-examine the situation carefully. It may be that the first prescription was mistaken, in which case the correct remedy must be prescribed. If, on the other hand, the diagnosis is confirmed, it is necessary to wait, unless there are well-founded suspicions that the remedy has been antidoted or is of poor quality.

The remedial action of the remedy will begin in proportion to the time it has taken to produce the symptoms in the proving.

Improper Action of the Remedy

The remedy may change the symptoms from inoffensive and painless to malignant and painful – for example, a rheumatism that damages the heart.

When the remedy changes the symptom picture and the patient's general state worsens, either the first prescription is only partially similar to the patient's totality, or else the disease is incurable.

If the disease is incurable, the remedial action of the drug must not be expected to be more than that of ameliorating symptoms, and the second prescription must be considered when new symptoms call for a new remedy.

If, after administering a remedy there are changes in the patient's symptoms without a general improvement, it must be acknowledged that the first prescription was mistaken, and that the true image of the disease has not been visualised.

It is then necessary to wait until the first symptom picture returns.

It is mistaken to prescribe a series of remedies for every changing symptom picture. The observant physician will know by the nature of the symptoms and the path they take whether the patient is improving or worsening, even though it may seem to the contrary to the patient or their family.

The first ailments may occur as symptoms change in the course of the patient's cure. If those symptoms are disturbed or palliated by a new prescription, the patient may definitely lose the possibility of being cured.

The purpose of the first prescription is to set the vital current on the appropriate path. Thus, the goal is the attainment of a psychic and organic equilibrium and a positive change in the patient's vital attitude. When negative factors which obstruct this healing current, such as hate, resentment, aggression, fears, dreads, anxiety and anguish are overcome – in other words, when mental symptoms disappear – a real cure is brought about. Nothing must interfere with this healing current; if it is hindered in any way, irreparable damage may be produced.

All this must be clearly discerned in a correctly drawn up clinical history, in such a way that the physician may examine the symptoms that disappear or reappear, and above all ascertain whether the patient is on the road to developing the ability to be positive and creative.

Chapter 12

Characterising the Symptom Picture
(1961)

In order to understand homoeopathy's position in modern medicine, the concept of chronic disease, and consequently what the physician must try to cure, must be fully grasped.

Clinical experience has convinced the modern physician that localised organic lesions are the final stage of a dysfunctional process which precedes pathological structure. At still deeper levels, we may find abnormal symptoms of susceptibility and reaction to the psychological and physical environment which make up the primary aspect of an individual's morbid predisposition.

Until the physician has therapeutically removed the original core of disease, he cannot rationally presume to have done anything to promote a real and profound cure in the patient. Moreover, if the physician has failed to perceive the patient as a biological unit and does not master the patient's constitutional predisposition, then he may at best suppress the patient's pathological symptoms without having understood the centrifugal releasing function of those symptoms.

Because life is a constant curative reaction, symptoms are simply exaggerated or perverted reactive phenomena. The abnormality of those vital reactions that turns them into symptoms depends on the individual's specific susceptibilities and genetic inheritance.

Under the generic name of psora, Hahnemann defined those abnormal susceptibilities which he considered to be the root of every morbid process. Psora dynamically conditions the psychic and functional behaviour of the child, still in a symbiotic relationship with the environment, and consequently determines the structure of his particular dysfunction or pathology.

Throughout a person's life, there are different factors linked to physiopathological reactive episodes. Although our character is genetically conditioned, different circumstances influence it to mould a unique personality, behaviour, social destiny, and therefore a unique pathological sequence.

An individual's personality or primary psychosomatic tendencies will always be present throughout their lifetime. Whether with few symptoms or many, latent or manifest, expressed in localised pathologies or camouflaged by strong defence mechanisms, this personality remains that individual's underlying dynamic predisposition.

The totality of the symptoms that characterise those reactions or primary susceptibilities – made manifest through a person's likes and dislikes, desires and aversions, habits, lifestyle and pathological and emotional accidents – yields a historical image of a dynamic process which no anatomical or pathological examination may parallel. No laboratory analysis can individualise a pathological symptom picture; at best, laboratory tests will offer only fragmentary aspects of a subject's whole economy. It is only through an individual's unique characteristic totality that one may obtain a clinical perspective of the real chronic disease.

Correct homoeopathic diagnosis, then, leads to a synthetic viewpoint of the clinical problem. Its goal is to cure the truly causal, constitutional elements of chronic disease – that is, the patient's reactive abnormality or maladjustment, not the repeated action of a germ or other alien force lodged in the organism as an incubus which must be expelled.

CASE 1

A 42-year-old radio technician had suffered from painful spasms in the right hypochondrium for twenty-six years.

He had been treated for his liver and gallbladder, amoebic parasites, appendicitis and allergies. He had undergone exploratory surgery in New York and was told he had something in his colon, though it was not certain what it was. He underwent many treatments to no avail. Often the colic spasms would come on after nervous excitement, arguments or worries. The painful cramps would subside a bit if he lay down on his back. Based on this, a prominent homoeopath prescribed Dioscorea. This patient's characteristic symptoms were:

Worse by milk
Worse by fruit
Worse fasting
Strong thirst
Perspiration of neck
Apathy
Bad temper
Anxiety

These symptoms, however, did not suffice to define clearly this patient's symptom picture. With common symptoms such as anxiety, apathy, bad temper and hysteria in the form of abdominal colic, I was as yet unable to define his type. But upon delving more deeply into his character, to my surprise, I found a man who felt a deep resentment against society. He was the youngest of five brothers and had been very spoiled by his father, who had died when he was fifteen. Following this he had to leave school in order to work. This first contact with the outside world, for which he was totally unprepared, unleashed a fiery rebelliousness against what he believed to be an unjust fate. Feeling as if he were being followed by enemies who tried to humiliate and vex him, he became obstinate and disobedient, refused to listen to any instructions from his supervisors and reacted to all constructive criticism with insults and cutting words.

This paranoid attitude and stubborn tendency to offend his supervisors meant that he failed to keep any job or position for long, even though he was successful at his work. His personality was composed of the following symptoms:

Reproaches others
Disobedience
Contemptuous
Desire to be alone
Worse by milk
Worse by fruit
Worse fasting
Thirst
Perspiration of neck

The repertorisation pointed directly to China, which has a paranoid personality with a marked tendency to insult and vex people. It was surprising to confirm how this patient changed his character after seven months of treatment; with three doses of China, two at 1M and one at 10M, the abdominal syndrome was completely cured and he turned into a placid and easygoing man who holds a steady job today in a private company.

CASE 2

A 49-year-old lawyer suffered from repeated bouts of bronchitis, asthma and a suppurating ear which had resisted every kind of treatment for thirty years. He also complained of boils in the groin and frequent styes on both eyelids. He was very nervous, irritable, excitable, sad, felt a desire to be alone, was averse to consolation and disliked people. He would start in his sleep, was very sensitive to cold, especially in the head and had a fetid foot-sweat.

His wife reported that just as he had to overcome his stubborn apathy and indifference, in order to come to my office again, she had to support him at all times so that he could practise his profession, because in the face of any difficulty he became easily disheartened and gave up the struggle. He was, however, very meticulous and conscientious in his work, going to abnormal extremes of anxiety and guilt about trivial details.

I was able to comprehend this man's symptom picture thanks to his wife's description, which revealed an obsessive and weak personality. His symptoms were the following:

Conscientious about trifles
Obstinate
Aggravated by consolation
Worse by cold
Sensitive to cold in head
Starting from sleep
Bromidrosis of feet

This syndrome is characteristic of Silica, which was his constitutional simillimum.

As in this case, Natrum Muriaticum has aggravation by consolation, but whereas Natrum Muriaticum rejects consolation with resentment and rage, Silica rejects consolation because, feeling inferior, it does not want anyone's pity.

A syndrome must be understood in terms of a personality, thus implying a characteristic totality and not an isolated phenomenon with no meaning in itself.

CASE 3

A 30-year-old single woman suffered from frequent boils and severe facial acne, for which she had undergone treatment with no success. Her symptom picture showed hot flushes, intolerance to the sun, to hot weather and to clothing on her chest and neck. She also felt a strong desire for ice-cold drinks, was easily bruised and suffered from an itchy scalp. There were no explicit mental symptoms.

Without repertorisation, Phosphorus was a remedy that came easily to mind, but her mental symptoms remained to be discovered. These usually come to the fore when the patient's lifestyle, family history and way of being are analysed. Her mother had died when she was ten years old, due to a fibroma. Physicians discovered that her mother had syphilis and thereupon decided to treat this patient with arsenic and bismuth for eight years. After her mother died she went to live with her aunt, to whom she was immensely attached, greatly affected by the anguish of her mother's death.

As the years went by, her aunt married and had two children. The patient's character then changed dramatically: she became sullen, aggressive and bad-tempered. Numerous boils and scabs appeared on her skin and she felt an intense aversion towards her aunt's children, which worsened to the point where her family life was unbearable. Undoubtedly, the jealousy was the determinative factor in her symptom picture, which also had aggravation by contact with clothing, hot flushes, desire for cold drinks, bruising and syphilis.

Phosphorus was excluded from this diagnosis. Uncontrollable jealousy determined Lachesis as the correct simillimum, even though Lachesis does not have the desire for cold drinks, which in this case was irrelevant in the face of her well-defined personality.

It is the characteristic totality that determines the therapeutic diagnosis of the simillimum, but that totality must always be defined by the personality and mental symptoms.

CASE 4

A 26-year-old single man had pyelonephritis symptoms for five months, with pains in the kidneys and bladder, polyuria with pyuria, a sub-feverish state, bleeding and painful haemorrhoids, great prostration, drowsiness, dry mucous membranes, irritability, bad temper and an intense fear of being alone, although at the same time he felt annoyed in the company of his family. Among the modalities and localised symptoms were nocturnal polyuria with great difficulty urinating, in spite of a constant urge to do so; great abdominal distension and much constipation with ineffectual urging and straining. A localised keynote symptom was a cold sensation in the penis. His mental symptoms were bad temper, irritability and a fear of being left alone, but at the same time rejecting other people's company to the point of not wanting anyone near him.

Lycopodium 30c and 200c completely removed the symptom picture in twenty days; however, he came back to my office a year and four months later with a strong burning sensation in the urethra on urinating, distended abdomen, constipation alternating with diarrhoea, burning sensation in the back and lumbar region, a foul foot-sweat he had had as a child and a strong desire for salty, spicy food.

I thought of Lycopodium, which had done him a lot of good before, but his mental symptom picture was not the same. This time he had a profound anxiety, a symptom which had been absent from the subacute episode of pyelonephritis. He did not fear being alone so much, but rather coming down with an incurable disease or being the victim of some terrible, inevitable disaster. He desperately wanted reassurance from his imagined dangers. His characteristic symptom picture, then, was the following:

Anxiety about future
Fear that something will happen
Desires highly seasoned food
Heat on back and lumbar region
Offensive foot perspiration

The indicated remedy was Phosphorus. When a patient's constitutional symptoms are concealed, the current symptom picture with the most recent symptoms must be treated. Later on, as the patient's true symptoms reappear and the case becomes clear, the constitutional background should be treated. This happens in practice and requires only that a physician know how to identify these symptoms.

CASE 5

A 50-year-old single woman came for a consultation. Three physicians had advised surgery to remove a fibroma the size of a grapefruit, which she wished to avoid.

She complained of indigestion, heartburn, nausea and chronic constipation. Hot weather and the sun caused headaches, but neither did she have much resistance against the cold. Her blood pressure was 200/130. She had no other physical symptoms. She lived with a married sister and felt a great affection for her 15-year-old nephew, having been a second mother to him. Apart from her nephew she had no close relationship with anyone; far from it, she felt a great aversion towards her brother-in-law and people in general, rejecting all social contact. She was sad, melancholic, depressed and pessimistic, tried to avoid people, and was extremely shy in front of strangers as well as people she knew. Strong headaches rendered her incapable of mental work. When she was thirty-six years old, her fiancé had abandoned her a month before the wedding, and thereafter she had become sad and

81

anxious with palpitations and trembling, all caused by the memory of the man who had betrayed her. Although she was an excellent concert pianist she was unable to sit at the piano and play, due to panic attacks that paralysed her.

The general and particular symptoms alone were insufficient to individualise her; it was only her life situation that had well-defined characteristics. The mental symptoms that she manifested in her behaviour, added to the few general symptoms and modalities, made up the following symptom picture:

Timidity
Aversion to members of family
Aversion to certain persons
Anxiety playing piano
Worse by warmth
Headache from exposure to sun
Indigestion

These seven symptoms clearly led to Natrum Carbonicum, which was administered in the 200c, 10M and 50M potencies, in several doses over a four-year period. Six years after her first consultation, and a full year taking nothing but a placebo, she has continued to come to my office because she has said she does not want to gain weight.

The fibroma has completely disappeared, her digestion is normal, she sleeps well and has no symptoms. She still lives with her sister and feels happy and content. Her relationships with friends and family are cordial. I believe that her fear of gaining weight lies in the fact that she is doing extremely well. She has a slender figure, admired by everyone (1.55 metres tall and weighing 55 kilograms) and does not want to lose her prestige now at the age of 56. She feels young, lively, strong, healthy, enthusiastic about life and, apart from a feeling of gratitude for her complete cure, the main reason she keeps coming to my office unnecessarily is her fear of losing these blessings.

A diagnosis must never be based on conjecture, deductions concerning physiopathological mechanisms, laboratory tests, or anything other than a clear and attentive study of the patient's functional psychological and physical symptoms.

Pathology cannot yield the elements necessary for individualisation, which can only be derived from the dynamic function of the personality. But to grasp the true mental symptoms, it is necessary to understand the totality of the patient's life circumstances, and to interpret this with logic and common sense, in order to discover authentic psychic reactions, and even general symptoms – seeing through the defensive camouflage which so often hides them.

We have seen Sepia, for example, hide her disaffection, loss of will-power and indifference and project her own aversion on to her spouse. Sepia says that it is her spouse who is cold and unloving and who wants to abandon her. As part of a primary self-defensive strategy, Sepia hides her sexual frigidity, the bearing-down sensation in the genital area and the signs that reveal her physical want of strength, whose moral conno-tation drives her to the edge of suicide – an idea she will never admit to harbouring as a relief from her loss of will-power. But the homoeopath will uncover the true psychological picture of a patient who bursts out crying in the consulting room unexpectedly, and who expresses more with her moans and countenance than with her words the enormous struggle to control her aggressive impulses, unacceptable to her con-science, directed against her husband and children, and the home from which she would like to escape and seek refuge in a hostile solitude devoid of consolation.

We have seen Arsenicum declare several times that she does not fear death in the least, but yet later confess timidly that she believes she will not be cured, that she has no salvation, that she has forebodings of death when alone, or that she will not survive an operation or any acute disease she may have.

We have seen Lycopodium hide stomach and liver symptoms, precisely because the troubles which produce a great anxiety in the epigastrium, generators of the cardinal symptoms of Lycopodium, were due to disagreements with his wife to whom he was attached, not daring to face his problem of neurotic dependency, conditioned by his chronic inferiority complex.

We could give many more examples which show the rigorous need, when prescribing, to characterise the symptom picture using a mini-mum of symptoms with a maximum value, in order to highlight the patient's personality.

Chapter 13

Finding the Simillimum
(1963)

To choose the simillimum which covers all the patient's essential characteristics, and sets the organism's vital curative reaction in motion, requires a philosophical perspective of the problem of humankind and disease.

The human being is not an animal, but a being with a moral conscience and a being who dies. When an animal dies it is extinguished, it simply disappears. Human beings do not live in terms of their animal nature, but in terms of a moral sense which impels them to develop their innate potential for transcendence. However, it is mistaken to consider the human being as a body subject to corruption and a spirit whose function is to conquer moral perfection. Just as the macrocosm fulfils its complete reproduction in the microcosm, the human being has been made the Divine image. As the Christian dogma of incarnation puts it, 'the word was made flesh'.

In human and moral life we assume our moral responsibility with our whole being, material and spiritual, body and soul. However, the unity of the human composite does not exclude the possibility that the spiritual soul may live without the body, or that, within certain limits, it may oppose the body. As the philosopher Max Scheler maintained, instinctive, passionate or psychosomatic forces are blind and chaotic, and yet without these instinctive forces the spirit is impotent.

Moral conscience is innate to the human being. In a battle with instinctive drives, moral conscience is thus capable of giving rise to mental and emotional symptoms such as anxiety, guilt, shame, fear, phobias, resentment and hate.

The homoeopath must base their clinical viewpoint on the patient's body-soul totality. Only then will they be able to integrate the symptoms which express that totality or essence.

The physician must understand that the patient's psychological state and moral conduct are the correlation of the physical problem. It is therefore no use for medicine to research physiopathological or physicochemical mechanisms if they are not referred directly to their fundamental cause, which resides in the mental stigma.

The stigmata of syphilis, tuberculosis and sycosis disturb the individual's instinctiveness. This in turn gives rise to psychological conflicts which interfere with normal vegetative functions. If the autonomic state is dysfunctional for too long a time, a pathological lesion may develop.

A patient's simillimum is the remedy diagnosed according to the particular mental and functional signs which express the totality of the individual as an inseparable body-soul unit.

Furthermore, it is not the function of homoeopathic remedies to correct organic or endocrinological dysfunctions, or humoral or physicochemical mechanisms, but to address the morbid susceptibility that stimulates and rectifies the vital force, in order to recover the organism's psychosomatic equilibrium. As Hahnemann maintained, this is achieved when the individual functions normally as a person, so that they may fulfil their highest ends of existence, which are none other than the development of their capacity for transcendence – or, according to depth psychology, the maturity of the personality.

Hahnemann's inspired perspective, as stated in the *Organon*, enables the homoeopath to rank the patient's symptoms and transfer the particular case to the materia medica. But to do this he or she must also master the art of repertorisation. Kent's *Repertory* is in strict conformity with the Hahnemannian idea of the patient, with a clinical schema which allows for individualisation from the mind to the organs, from general to particular symptoms, from the individual's centre of vital activity – their instinctiveness, desires and aversions, likes and dislikes – to the particular modalities, down to the last details of their system. A correct repertorisation will mirror the whole human being, complete in the essence of that individual's particular characteristic symptoms.

The symptoms gathered from remedy provings are exclusive to homoeopathy and allow for the individualisation of the patient. Homoeopathic diagnoses deductively arrived at by way of pathological symptoms, or comparisons with similar previous cases, are not consistent with authentic homoeopathy. The proving symptoms are part of the dynamic process that precedes any changes in tissue structure. None of the remedies from the materia medica has been proven to the point of producing tissue damage. A symptom cured by a remedy is the clinical verification of black type in the *Repertory*. However, Kent was careful to exclude any clinical symptoms which contradicted symptoms from the provings.

Pathologists who seek the remedy capable of producing an ulcer, pneumonia or sciatica would do well to bear in mind that these affections are nevertheless modified in the patient by different modalities, and that it is precisely in these modalities that the individualisation of each case of ulcer, pneumonia or sciatica lies.

After reviewing a patient's complete clinical history, the homoeopath must attempt to discover that person's particular idiosyncrasy. This is accomplished only after distinguishing between:

(i) the pathognomonic symptoms which correspond to the current disease;

(ii) the common symptoms shared by many patients and many remedies at the same time, such as anxiety, fears, uneasiness, headaches, weakness, and other symptoms which make up the general rubrics in the repertory;

(iii) the characteristic symptoms which really define the patient as a particular case. These characteristic symptoms, the only symptoms capable of leading the physician to a correct diagnosis, are beyond classification or physiopathological interpretation.

Characteristic or peculiar symptoms may be found in the three great groups of mental, general or particular symptoms – understanding by particular symptoms those which refer to parts of the body.

These three great groups determine the rubrics that refer to symptoms in general and are registered in the thirty-seven sections of the repertory. When a rubric or general symptom includes many remedies, it is a common symptom and therefore not useful for repertorisation. However, each rubric or general symptom is modified by the following six factors:

(i) sides;

(ii) time;

(iii) conditions, circumstances, etc.;

(iv) extending;

(v) localisation

(vi) character.

It is in these modifications of general symptoms, hereby transformed into particular symptoms, that the patient's peculiar characteristic symptoms will be found. (Here the word 'particular' refers to the particularisation of the symptom and not to parts of the body.) Often, when clearly marked and belonging to one or two remedies, a rare, strange and peculiar symptom will be discovered – a true keynote of the case.

A correct repertorisation is an artistic endeavour in which the homoeopath's skills come into play. Science informs the physician about homoeopathic doctrine, but clinical practice also requires good artistic faculties to apply this doctrine and get a sound case history.

The homoeopath chooses three or four essential characteristic symptoms: either strange, rare and peculiar symptoms which cannot be explained by any pathological process, or common general and mental symptoms, modified by one or more of the six factors mentioned above.

If the homoeopath is sure of the first two characteristic symptoms that determine the case, he has only to cross-reference them in order to identify the remedies that are present in both, thus reducing the list of remedies to those which agree.

For the final selection of the remedy, the simillimum must be present in this small list, which in turn must be compared with the rest of the symptom picture.

One 63-year-old man derived enormous benefits from a remedy which provoked a marked aggravation with the return of old catarrhal discharges through the bronchial tubes. He suffered from emphysema, asthma, rheumatism, dyspepsia and polyuria, as well as a nervous excitable state with excessive fastidiousness concerning insignificant details of daily life. Not only did he reproach his family for every little thing, but he was easily irked and rejected the least hint of affection from his wife and daughters. He suffered from fatigue and precordial oppression, and every night he would moan 'Ah ... Ah!' in his sleep, which made his family suppose he was suffering terribly.

The only symptom this man complained of was a constricting sensation in his chest, as if he were wrapped by a tight band around the thorax. The other symptoms he had, such as a sensitivity to cold, perspiration, rheumatic pains and gastrointestinal ailments were common symptoms without particular modalities. His blood pressure was 200/110 and his heart was in good condition.

Associating, as determinative characteristic symptoms, 'Moaning during sleep' and 'Chest constriction as from a band', the matching remedies in both rubrics are Arsenicum, Bryonia, Lycopodium, Opium and Silica. Completing the repertorisation with the two characteristic mental symptoms: 'Fastidious' and 'Aggravation by consolation', Arsenicum was clearly the remedy. Without this repertorisation, which led to an exact diagnosis, I would not have been able to pinpoint Arsenicum as the remedy for a patient who hid and denied his fear of death behind the façade of a gloomy and rude character who hated consolation.

Another patient, a 41-year-old man, had had asthma for fifteen years, with chronic rhinitis and bronchitis together with a vague anxiety that would set him on the edge of despair. He was unable to establish the motives, nature or modalities of his anxiety; however, backed up by his family, he stated that he found relief only by being busy, whether in his work or at any manual task into which he could throw himself whole-heartedly. He had a real need to be busy at something, not only to calm his anxiety, but to assuage his irritability when in contact with people. His sensitivity to cold would come to the fore when he exposed some part of his body, when he took off his warm wraps, or even when he undressed at night, which would immediately bring on bouts of sneez-ing. He also had indigestion, constipation, profuse perspiration during sleep and a slight rise in his temperature during the evening, all of these being common symptoms with no special modalities except for a marked hourly aggravation of the asthmatic crises and the anxiety at 3 a.m.

Cross-referencing the mental symptoms 'Amelioration by occupa-tion', 'Occupation, amel.', 'Industrious' and 'Busy', with the physical symptoms 'Aggravation after a part of the body becoming cold', 'Aggravation uncovering' and 'Aggravation undressing' points to Baryta Carbonica, Belladonna, Sepia, Rhus Tox. and Silica. Of these five remedies, the only one which worsens after 3 a.m. is Sepia, which was this patient's remedy.

One dose of Sepia 200c provoked an intense aggravation forty-eight hours later, which took the form of a bad asthma attack. However, this time, his asthma was accompanied by fever and a copious bronchial catarrh. Because his family feared he had bronchopneumonia, a phys-ician was summoned. This physician, being a homoeopath, thought the symptom picture fitted Antimonium Tartaricum but, after having been informed of my prescription, decided upon a placebo. The next day, everything had subsided except for a profuse elimination which took the form of a tracheobronchial catarrh, an old symptom he had had years before, when his ailment had begun.

Two or three weeks later, he was completely free of his asthma symptoms and he completely recovered from his anxiety, irritability and fatigue. Three months later, another dose of Sepia 200c immedi-ately cured an asthmatic cold which he developed.

The diagnosis of this case was based on two characteristic determin-ative symptoms: amelioration by occupation and aggravation after a part of the body becoming cold, which cross-referenced his other symptoms.

A patient's clinical history usually contains three or four determinative symptoms which refer to the unique way in which he reacts as a whole living unit. Depending on the patient, these symptoms may be mental, general or have particular modalities. If the physician is capable of detecting these few symptoms – and not merely identifying localised pains and inflammations – he is on the road to a precise diagnosis.

The homoeopath must know how to modify or particularise common mental, general or particular symptoms. What pragmatically ranks a symptom as characteristic is not its value as an isolated symptom, but its integration with other general symptoms.

Mental symptoms categorically define a symptom picture. Thus, when mental and general symptoms are clearly marked in a patient, they eliminate any particular symptoms which might also be present. Similarly, clearly marked mental symptoms cancel out any general symptoms which do not agree. On the other hand, a general symptom must always be covered by the mental condition for which it has value.

A 75-year-old woman suffered from chronic deformative rheumatism with intense pains that worsened considerably during thunderstorms. This was confirmed by her children, who accompanied her to my office.

In the absence of thunderstorms her pains were less, but nevertheless permanent. Her family observed that when she was entertained or occupied at something, she forgot her pains and was calm, but if anybody asked her about her problems she immediately felt them again. She admitted herself that when she paid attention to her ailments, her pains reasserted themselves.

An essential characteristic mental symptom of hers, then, was aggravation upon thinking of her pains.

She also had great physical restlessness with vague and imprecise fears, polyuria, incontinence, great heat and a burning sensation in her feet which made her uncover them at night.

With these clearly marked characterisations, I drew up the following repertorisation:

Extremities, pain, thunderstorm agg.	Med., Nat. c., Rhod.
Thinking, complaints of, agg.	Med.
Heat, foot burning	Med.

After a tolerable aggravation which took the form of diarrhoea and polyuria – which no doubt helped to eliminate a great deal of toxins – the improvement which this patient felt with a single dose of Medorrhinum 10M was extraordinary.

Based on the heat and aggravation during thunderstorms, but ignoring the mental condition, this woman had been previously treated with Rhododendron 1M and Sulphur 1M.

Mental symptoms are not restricted to conscious psychological expressions or a person's behaviour. Mental symptoms are classified as symptoms of the will, intelligence, emotions and memory. Symptoms pertaining to the will refer to instinctive tendencies that determine desires and aversions regarding a person's relationship with life and fellow human beings, or even desires and aversions linked to our instinct for preservation – of our own selves or of our species – such as food preferences and sexuality. Our instinctiveness is grounded in the unconscious will that emerges from the innermost depths of our being, where vital energy presides over metabolic changes in the cell and structures our psychophysical personality.

The centre of the morbid process is always to be found in the patient's instinctiveness. This expresses itself not only in emotional symptoms, but also in their desires and aversions, in sexual and menstrual derangements, and because food and emotions travel through the digestive tract, in a disturbed appetite and gastrointestinal dysfunction. Of less value are symptoms of the intelligence, such as mental confusion or an inability to concentrate, and a faulty memory.

Because mental symptoms are frequently hidden behind a defensive mask, the physician must often divert his attention from the patient's emotional state and behaviour to focus on the physical derangements that have resulted from the patient's unconscious will.

A correct clinical history, and in some cases reports from the patient's relatives, will shed light on the patient's emotional state. Nevertheless, instinctive disturbances are not only capable of turning into psychic symptoms, but into systemic dysfunctions as well.

All the general symptoms, such as reactions to changes in climate, desires for and aversions to food, perspiration, activity, sexuality, dreams, periodicity, bleeding, abnormal tissue repair and discharges, secretions and excretions, come from emotional disturbances which express a certain way of being. As is frequently observed, an emotion may even bring about a special odour in perspiration or impart a special trait to any secretion.

A 31-year-old woman came to my office. She was a mother of three, one child being retarded as a result of encephalitis at the age of one. She suffered from burning pains in the stomach, a sensation of epigastric sluggishness, fullness after eating, pains in the right hypochondrium which radiated to the back, constipation which alternated with diarrhoea, great mental and physical fatigue, extreme irritability and intolerance, bouts of weeping with a sensation of impotence, attacks of vertigo, and numbness in the hands and legs. During her last pregnancy, a year and a half previously, she had come down with hepatitis and a recent laboratory test showed a great number of amoebic parasites. Her emotional state revolved around her retarded son, against whom she had developed a deep resentment. Aggressive, stubborn and jealous, this child manipulated his mother through his whims and constant demands for attention.

The woman felt mortified by what she felt to be a terribly unjust fate. She bemoaned her misfortune and rejected bitterly every attempt to console her. This state of intolerance, bitterness and despair took the form of a true anxiety neurosis, and she underwent treatment with a competent psychoanalyst who, after two years of therapy, was able to make her understand her abnormal relationship with her son, in the light of her own resentments and frustrations with her parents and spouse. However, the psychoanalyst was unable to obtain any radical change in her attitude, or any improvement in her general physical state of sluggishness and nervousness. It was then, as a last resort, that she turned to homoeopathy.

In keeping with our rule of strictly adhering to symptoms, avoiding any conjecture concerning mental attitudes which are not clearly explicit, it was nevertheless clear that this patient felt an aversion towards her son, as in Lycopodium, Platinum and Sepia. Thus I construed her symptom picture.

She craved sweets to the point of preferring to eat desserts and chocolate instead of lunch or dinner, which her family always found peculiar.

The menses were brown, a fact confirmed by her mother.

All her symptoms, especially the irritability, tiredness and pains in the waist, were aggravated by wet weather. Her general state was significantly worse in the spring, to the point of bringing on a general prostration.

More than at any other time of day, she felt extremely weak on rising in the morning. After defecating she felt a painful, anxious sensation in the abdomen with much restlessness and a vague, inexplicable fear.

The perspiration was profuse and offensive, the breath was foul, the abdomen was distended and painful, the blood pressure was 110/90, and the ankles were swollen with an obstructed vein.

By cross-referencing the following two main characteristic symptoms, 'Desires sweets' with 'Menses brown', we obtain the following remedies which agree with both rubrics: Bryonia, Calcarea Carbonica, Carbo Vegetabilis, Rhus Tox., Secale and Sepia, which also share 'Aggravation by spring'. Continuing with the repertorisation, 'Aggravation by wet weather' is shared by Bryonia, Calcarea Carbonica, Carbo Vegetabilis, Rhus Tox and Sepia. 'Anxiety, abdomen, after stool' is present only in Sepia and 'Weakness, morning on rising' is shared by Bryonia and Sepia.

Sepia, then, not only emerged from the repertorisation, but covered the totality of the patient's symptoms of debility, sluggishness, tiredness, irritability, fastidiousness, intolerance, indifference and venous stasis.

A first dose of Sepia 200c caused an aggravation with insomnia, an increase of leucorrhoea and an anal itch, after which her symptom picture remained stationary for some time. Two months later, Sepia 1M brought about an eczema on the face and neck. Forty days later, because her physical and moral apathy had not changed to any significant degree in spite of her general improvement, I prescribed Sepia 10M.

A few days after this last dose, she radically changed her attitude regarding her son, entrusting his care to a special institution. Because of the masochistic feelings related to the resentment that she felt towards this child, whom she blamed for her misfortune, she had refused to take this step before. Thereafter her character softened noticeably. She became calm, patient, affectionate and devoted towards this son, her other two children and her husband. Never again did she curse her fate.

Two years of psychoanalysis and conventional medication had not modified her mental state; although she had come to understand the nature of her relationship with her son on the analyst's couch, she had not been cured of the emotional disturbance that made her reject him, going against her maternal instincts. Only Sepia was able to do that.

This case illustrates the fact that what a patient loves and hates – the innermost core of their emotional life – has its correlation in the desires and aversions of instinctive needs. This woman's abnormal desire for sweets and the peculiar colour of her menses were a physical expression of the anguish she felt.

Thus, aside from any conjectures or clinical deductions, it is important to take note of the symptoms that express the patient as a vital unit, whether they be general symptoms or particular modalities.

In homoeopathy, it is the person, not the disease, that is of interest to the physician. In keeping with current psychosomatic thought, symptoms which express a patient's functioning are not only in the mind, as classical psychology contends, but also in the whole body.

A characteristic symptom may be a modality of a particular symptom, or simply a symptom which appears to be unrelated to the syndrome that corresponds to the organic or localised disease.

These apparently isolated symptoms are considered 'strange, rare and peculiar'. Guernsey called them keynote symptoms because they 'opened' the case. Even though they are particularities of localised symptoms and do not appear to be general symptoms which represent the patient's totality, because they are not pathognomonic to the localised disease, they nevertheless do most certainly belong to the patient and not to the disease.

However, physicians must guard against considering keynote symptoms in an isolated fashion and basing their prescriptions on them. General symptoms and the patient's mental condition must agree with keynote symptoms and not contradict them. To suppress a symptom does not mean that a patient is cured; cure is achieved only when all symptoms are eradicated.

A 54-year-old woman had been advised to undergo surgery for a stomach ulcer. She also suffered from burning pains in the stomach after eating, as well as rheumatic pains in the large joints, with no modalities. She was worse by cold and in the open air, had a profuse and offensive foot-sweat, tiredness with no modalities, a vaginal itch and perineal eczema.

All her symptoms were common and did not lead to a specific characterisation. However, after being asked to give details on her behaviour and any peculiar sensations she felt, she admitted that she had involuntary urination on putting her hands in cold water, which is covered only by Kreosotum. This was a true keynote symptom which needed to agree with the rest of the symptoms. Kreosotum is aggravated by the cold and open air, has a profuse foot-sweat, vaginal itch, eczema between folds of the skin and burning pains in the stomach after eating. Her teeth had dark stains on them which her dentist attributed to the iodised water of the country village where she had lived before, but she said that her relatives and other inhabitants of that same village did not have such stains on their teeth.

Kent's *Repertory* has 'Teeth discolored, dark in spots', covered only by Kreosotum. This is no happy coincidence, but the clinical verification, based on an ordinary case, that particular modalities and peculiar symptoms express a symptom picture with a special harmonious correlation which goes far beyond the disease picture. If the physician has not been able to find the patient's characteristic symptoms, or rare, strange and peculiar symptoms, and does not perform a detailed repertorisation that reveals the patient's idiosyncrasy, he or she will not be able to attain the strict individualisation that is necessary. Intuition can never take the place of repertorisation, which often yields surprising results.

In this case, I never would have thought of Kreosotum if it had not been for the keynote symptoms, corroborated, of course, by the general symptoms. One dose of Kreosotum 1M followed by another dose of Kreosotum 10M three months later cured her of her stomach ulcer, thus making surgery unnecessary.

Deductions concerning physiopathological mechanisms prevent the orthodox physician from understanding the relationship between the psychological or functional symptom and tissue damage. However, clinical evidence is always to be preferred over any deductive system. The true homoeopath responds only to a rigorous examination of the facts, that is, the symptoms, which allow him to observe in clinical reality the theoretical formulation of the psychosomatic unity of the morbid process.

The following case bears eloquent witness to the drama that may be wrought in patients as a result of the stubborn application of criteria alien to mental factors.

A mother brought her 17-year-old daughter to my office. The girl had a persistent fever which had begun six months before when, on coming home from school, she felt faint, had colic with no bowel movements and developed a fever which climbed to 40°C that evening. The physician who was summoned diagnosed acute appendicitis. She was given antibiotics and underwent an appendectomy the next day. Her fever continued at 39°C and 39.5°C, in spite of the operation and subsequent treatment.

Three or four weeks later, because her feverish state, her general breakdown and stomach pains had not subsided, she underwent X-ray and laboratory tests which revealed cholesterol accumulations in her gallbladder. This patient had never felt pains in her liver nor her hypochondrium, and the radiologist himself did not believe that the presence of soft stones in her gallbladder – which was not inflamed nor even irritated – could be the cause of her temperature.

In spite of the fact that a precise diagnosis had not been arrived at, it was decided to remove her gallbladder four months after her appendectomy. Once out of the operating room, the doctor who performed surgery on this girl, no doubt on seeing that her gallbladder was healthy and that the gallstones were of no consequence, told her mother that the fever would continue. Indeed, the girl's previous state did not change at all, except for a slow decline in her vitality. She was heavily dosed with antibiotics to no avail, except for chloromycetin, which for a few days managed to bring her temperature down to 37.8°C in the morning, only to have it rise to 39°C again in the evening. Two months after this operation, as a last resort, the family turned to homoeopathy.

The clinical history began with the first moments of this girl's symptom picture, which had begun six months before when she had taken a history examination. She had completed her fourth year at business school, and history was a required third-year subject which she was lacking. It was imperative that she passed this examination because she would not otherwise be able to proceed to the fifth year. She went to take her exam in a terrible state of anxiety, having to wait for a long time for her name to be called. She reported that, while the board of examiners retained one classmate for fifty minutes, she was in the examination room for no more five minutes. While this classmate passed the exam, she failed it because they asked her only two questions and she was able to answer only one satisfactorily. She thought her classmate had been treated favourably because she was related to one of the teachers on the examination board – she felt great indignation at this, along with spasms in her stomach and a desire to vomit, all of which caused her to run home. Hours later, her temperature rose. It was then that an appendectomy was decided on.

This patient's current symptom picture revealed an extreme change in her character. During the interview, the girl was reticent and hostile. Her mother, who told the story, assured me that from the day of the examination and the appendectomy which immediately followed, her daughter's mood had changed drastically. Usually kind and cheerful, she became bitter, irritable, sad, abusive and hostile towards her family, friends and people in general. Not only did she reject people, wishing to be left alone, but she became very indignant at the slightest attempt to console her or cheer her up.

Her symptom picture was as follows: tiredness with general lethargy, especially at mid-morning; feverish state peaking at 38.5°–39°C in the early afternoon; intense thirst with a variable appetite; her favourite food was coffee with milk, bread and sweets; persistent pains in the epigastrium with a convulsive constriction of the stomach, with the characteristic symptom that before eating her lunch, afternoon snack or dinner, she felt great drowsiness and often had to sleep for a few minutes. Her drowsiness was apparently caused by hunger and never came up at any other time of day.

In order to perform the repertorisation, I cross-referenced two determinative characteristic symptoms: 'Aggravation by consolation' with 'Ailments after anger, vexation, etc.'. I preferred this larger rubric to the smaller 'Ailments after anger with indignation' in order to avoid the possibility of losing the remedy. The other characteristic symptoms were 'Sleepiness before eating' and 'Constriction, convulsive, in stomach'.

These four determinative symptoms clearly led to Natrum Muriaticum, a remedy easily perceived from my first impressions, but diagnosed with certainty and precision after the repertorisation.

A single dose of Natrum Muriaticum 1M provoked in this patient an intense but tolerable headache, followed by a spectacular improvement, with the eradication of her fever and swift recovery. Her character and behaviour changed radically and even the colour in her face improved, to the astonishment of her family. Her fever did not recur, she came out of her shell, resumed her studies and today, five months after the first consultation, is perfectly well, having required only one more dose of Natrum Muriaticum 1M to treat a constrictive sensation in the epigastrium.

I cannot understand what clinical criteria led this patient to such large doses of antibiotics and two unnecessary operations. Only dogmatic thought can approve of medical practices which identify fever with a microbial infection, oblivious of the fact that fever reactions are determined by thermogenic centres of the brain, disturbed, in this case, by an emotional shock.

Even though the apparent cause or provoking factor of the current symptom picture may count as a determinative symptom in the patient's basic symptom picture, it must never be considered as the only symptom that can guide to the diagnosis of the simillimum.

Moreover, it is often necessary to face situations in daily practice in which the patient does not appear to have characteristic symptoms on which to base a diagnosis. Hahnemann called these cases 'defective diseases', in which the modalities of the current symptom picture or localised disease prevail, thus masking the patient's constitutional symptomatology. This may occur, for example, in acute states in which it is sometimes necessary to administer the remedy which corresponds to the current condition.

The current state may be the consequence of an acute disease triggered by infection, emotional trauma, physical injury or intoxication by drugs. In these cases, the homoeopath must identify the remedy that matches the current symptom picture, which will often make constitutional symptoms reappear, thus providing a firm basis for the diagnosis of the simillimum. But even if this were impossible to do, the physician may turn to those remedies which clear the case or which antidote the causal factor that brought about the current condition. In such cases, the physician may choose a remedy which would have corresponded to the initial moments of the symptom picture, a nosode of the acute ailment, or a stimulator of nervous energy.

Futhermore, in the rubrics 'Lack of reaction', 'Lack of irritability' and 'Sluggishness of the body' we may find the circumstantial remedy for those cases, all too frequent nowadays, whereby the patient's reactive sensitivity has been obstructed or deranged by medication with tranquillisers, corticosteroids, vitamins, antibiotics etc. and in which it is impossible to discern the true symptoms of the disease.

In any case, when the remedy matches the case, it will antidote the effects from drugs, acute infections or emotional factors.

Remedy provings have not been performed on many nosodes. Unless prescribed in accordance with homoeopathic criteria – that is, strictly matching the patient's symptoms – nosodes can never take the place of the simillimum which reflects the patient.

Foubister reintroduced Carcinosin into homoeopathic clinical practice, advising that symptoms should be carefully analysed before using it, as in any nosode.

Carcinosin's symptom picture is briefly summarised as follows:

These young patients are restless; excitable; with a marked insomnia; a tendency to sleep in the genupectoral position (as in Muslim prayer) like Medorrhinum, Tuberculinum, Phosphorus, Calcarea Phosphorica, Sepia and Lycopodium or with their hands over their heads, as in Pulsatilla. They are meticulous, neat and tidy, as opposed to Sulphur; stubborn as in Tuberculinum; noted for their sense of rhythm and fondness for dancing, as in Sepia; precocious and gifted, understanding more than what is expected of them at their age (one 2-year-old girl spontaneously discovered a woman's 6-month pregnancy and asked her mother why she too did not have that 'belly'); affectionate and congenial as in Phosphorus; very sensitive to contradiction or reprimands as in Medorrhinum; fearful and apprehensive before certain events; crave fat and sweets. Persistently anorexic children will crave sweets to the point of not wanting to eat anything except sugar.

One 10-year-old boy came to my office with asthma and bronchitis. His mother reported that the boy had had measles at the age of 1fi and that then he had suffered from his lung ailment. Before the measles, he had been in perfect health.

These facts, which attributed his asthma and bronchitis to the measles, could easily have led to the prescription of Morbillinum; however, the boy had other symptoms.

He would soak the pillow every night with a profuse and fetid perspiration. He also had goose flesh with tiny scabs on the skin, making it dry and rough. He was extremely shy with strangers and contrary, opposing any suggestion offered to him.

I considered the fetid head-sweat as the determinative symptom and construed the symptom picture as follows:

Perspiration, scalp, fetid	Calc. Carb., Merc., Puls., Staph.
Perspiration, scalp, sleep, during	Calc. Carb., Merc.
Gooseflesh	Calc. Carb., Merc.
Timidity	Calc. Carb., Merc.
Contradict, disposition to	Merc.

Mercurius was the remedy for this boy, who also had serious behaviour problems. He constantly looked for fights, was extremely irritable to the point of wanting to kill the person who contradicted him, and always opposed any suggestion offered to him. This tendency to contradict was the characteristic symptom which favoured Mercurius over Calcarea. Mercurius is the only remedy in 'Desire to kill the person who contradicts her'. The larger rubrics 'Quarrelsome' and 'Wants to fight' were eliminated from the repertorisation because they were unnecessary.

A single dose of Mercurius 1M produced a dry, scaly skin eruption on both palms, similar to a post-scarlatinal peeling, a profuse nasal catarrh and a fetid foot-sweat which his mother said he had had when he was very small but which had later gone away spontaneously. His behaviour changed radically. His aggressiveness and negative attitude disappeared completely, as well as his asthma and bronchitis.

The patient's mental and psychological condition should be the first requirement before ranking the symptoms and determining the diagnosis. As long as patients do not modify their mental state they are not healing, but rather suppressing organic or pathological expressions which may, for example, lead to an irreversible metastasis or to the definite fixation of a neurosis.

A 3-year-old boy was brought to my office with a severe eczema all over his body. His father, a physician, had given him all the homoeopathic remedies usually prescribed for eczema in children: Sulphur, Calcarea Carbonica, Sepia, etc.

The child's skin eruption had all the common modalities of Sulphur – an intense itch aggravated by the heat of the bedclothes at night; great restlessness and irritability when walking in the open air; intense thirst during meals and intolerance of bathing. The father asked why Sulphur had not acted in spite of having been administered at several different potencies.

His son's characteristic symptoms were: 'Irritability in children'; 'Obstinate'; 'Capriciousness'; 'Aggravated by warm wraps'; 'Aggravated by warmth of bed'; and 'Desires cold drinks'.

Repertorisation in this case led to Chamomilla. Among others, Sulphur and Calcarea were last on the list. A dose of Chamomilla 200c improved the child's condition immensely from the first night; his eczema started to subside three weeks later. The following month I gave him another dose of Chamomilla 200c and two months later he came to my office completely cured of his eczema. This persistent eruption had begun on a spot on his right forearm two years before; it was also the last spot to be clear of the eruption. He stopped being irritable, stubborn and capricious.

Although he seemed to be in good health, there was something peculiar about his demeanour that I observed during subsequent consultations. He was always by his mother's side, kissing her constantly and seeking to be petted and caressed. His parents reported that their son was now extremely sensitive and affectionate. He loved being touched, rubbed or caressed on his abdomen, head, or any other part of his body which he claimed hurt.

He had developed a symptom which is made up of three rubrics in the repertory: 'Ameliorated by rubbing'; 'Desires to be magnetised'; and 'Ameliorated by magnetism'.

This young patient, then, had suppressed his psoric release. Although Chamomilla had been correctly prescribed it was not his true simillimum, but only a remedy similar to the current symptom picture, just as the occasional remedy may be similar to an acute disease. I felt that the boy was expressing the first symptoms of his latent pseudo-psora in the form of an extreme sensitivity to being petted and the magnetic influence of caresses, and that, because Chamomilla had not been able to rouse his true symptomatology enough, perhaps he actually needed an acute infection in order to bring out the constitutional remedy. Three years after the eczema disappeared, he contracted angina with a high fever which lasted six days. Two months later his parents reported that he had been very frightened, not only by a thunderstorm, but also by an imminent storm which never materialised but just blew over. Before the angina, he was afraid of thunderstorms, but never as afraid as after the angina. He also sweated profusely upon falling asleep, and had acquired the habit of eating cold food to the point of asking for his food directly from the refrigerator. As a seemingly trivial corollary, his parents added that he always liked to be clean and tidy, taking extra care to wear clean shoes and be impeccably dressed.

'Fear of thunderstorm' with 'Perspiration on beginning to sleep' are shared by Mercurius, Phosphorus, Sepia and Sulphur. Of these four remedies, only Phosphorus has a desire for cold food. After this brief repertorisation, I decided Phosphorus was his constitutional remedy. Phosphorus covered his extreme sensitivity, affection, tidiness, daintiness and need for consolation, caresses and massage, equivalent to the desire to be magnetised. After taking Phosphorus, this young patient's general state changed considerably. He gained weight, changed his demeanour and is now developing normally. His eczema did not return because Chamomilla had completed a cycle of psoric release, which remained latent until a new acute episode aroused the symptoms which brought his simillimum to the fore once again.

In spite of the healing function of acute diseases and elimination crises, chronic disease is never cured of its own accord. Only the simillimum may do this, when it fulfils the law of similarity between the characteristic pathogenic symptoms, which define the healing power of the remedy, and the characteristic symptoms of the patient, which define what must be cured.

Through the art of repertorisation, the homoeopath must carefully scrutinise mental and general symptoms as well as the particularities of common and local symptoms in each case, in order to assess the patient properly as an untold and indivisible body-soul unit, and thus to find the curative simillimum.

Chapter 14

The Practice of Homoeopathy I
(1957)

Only an insubstantial understanding of medicine, and ignorance of the medical ideas that lend support to homoeopathy, can give rise to doubts concerning its validity. Renewed by contemporary clinical theory and practice, homoeopathic theory has had life since the publication of Hahnemann's *Organon* in 1810. When practised according to its original principles, homoeopathy is an amazing verification of Hippocratic medicine's foremost claim – the individualisation of each clinical form of disease. Unfortunately, much of the homoeopathy practised today lacks the Hahnemannian spirit.

Homoeopathy is a therapeutic technique based on experiments with drugs performed on human beings and on an inductive theory of chronic disease, all of which give rise to three basic principles: (i) the single remedy, (ii) the similar remedy and (iii) the minimum dose.

Prescriptions are based exclusively on the totality of symptoms. Patients are characterised by ranking their symptoms as: (i) mental symptoms, (ii) aggravations and improvements, (iii) likes and dislikes, (iv) general symptoms and (v) particular symptoms.

The diagnosis based on pathological syndromes is replaced with a new diagnosis based on the similarity between natural syndromes and the syndromes produced by drug provings performed on relatively healthy human beings. The symptom picture produced by each drug yields its pathogenesis, which the physician later applies by analogy. This therapeutic diagnosis involves everything that medical knowledge can glean as signs of how human beings react to pathogenic or injurious agents. In this way, information on the symptom pictures recorded in the drug provings is expanded. Thus homoeopathy is not dogmatic or deficient. Still relevant, however, is the collection of subjective and objective symptoms that were proved by Hahnemann and his followers – the most original and detailed transcription of reactive symptoms directly experienced by human beings.

Homoeopathy turns to all branches of medicine which may help it to make pathological, neurological and psychological diagnoses. However, although these are of value, they do not determine the therapeutic diagnosis in homoeopathy. Also, common symptoms are set apart from the patient's unique characteristic symptoms.

Homoeopathy's indispensable requirement is to individualise each case; that is, to discover each patient's personal quotient. Cutting across quantitative determinism, each patient presents variations of the syndrome or morbid process. It may be said that homoeopathy, above and beyond a classificatory system of concepts for generic diseases, is a subjective system of symptoms for each particular case.

It is the physician's task to comprehend the patient's whole psychosomatic symptom picture. To prescribe homoeopathic remedies that address symptoms in isolation from their integrating function in the patient's life history is to transgress homoeopathy's holistic principles.

An inflamed throat can be cured with antibiotics, localised medication, homoeopathic remedies or with no medication at all. However, this nullification does not mean that the case has been solved, nor does it prevent relapses or metastases of the constitutional morbid process which underlies the inflammation and conditions the terrain for acute crises. An indiscriminate suppression of symptoms, divorced from the patient's life history and general context, courts failure.

To intoxicate an organism with drugs is not the only way to assault it. Whether with massive or minimum doses, the greatest aggression that any therapeutic system can commit is to suppress symptoms and expressions which should have been respected. They may sometimes be vicarious, at other times meaningful integrating factors of a vital unit, but they always perform a releasing and necessary function.

The physician is not an arbitrator who interferes in the healing process of nature, but a helper who knows what must be corrected or activated in the spontaneous play of vital reactions. Thus, the physician guides each patient to redirect his natural course of life and assess whether he needs to correct his diet, reshape his circumstances, resolve a conflict, relieve a tension or even address an organic or localised affection with physical procedures, surgery, psychotherapy or medication. Homoeopathy is not above such practices as applying several remedies at one time as a temporary measure. But the homoeopath must never forget that such temporary measures are no more than palliative treatment that prevents a real knowledge of the patient, and thus the opportunity to influence the law of cure.

Vital phenomena are meaningful inasmuch as they are processes which further the attainment of an individual's personal goals. It is here that ideas grounded in an honest desire to help are to be found and where all medical thought converges as one.

The Hahnemannian concept of chronic disease as a dynamic process that conditions the somatic state, structures the functional system and moulds the personality, has been distorted by a form of homoeopathy which considers disease to be a blockage due to toxins, a dysfunctional organ or a physical inability to adapt. The Hahnemannian concept of pyschophysical totality has been replaced by that of an aggregate of organs and functions which may be repaired in an isolated fashion or drained of toxins, disregarding the fact that these dynamic disturbances are actually rooted in the patient's constitutional personality.

This is only to be expected if the homoeopath adheres to organic criteria concerning disease and is unable to acknowledge that the laws of the individual can modify or replace the laws of physiological mechanics. General symptoms such as debility, insomnia, sensitivity to cold and so on, or symptoms which Hahnemann called 'strange, rare and peculiar', are all reactive phenomena that go beyond the more or less autonomous circuit of the physiological mechanism. The meaning of such symptoms are subject to the totality of the individual, and can only be expressed in psychological terms.

The constitution is the personality, and the personality is that which is psychological. However, it must be understood that for Hahnemann, as in modern clinical practice, there are no ailments which are solely psychological or solely physical in origin. That which is psychological or mental is no more than a special type of biological reaction. There is no such thing as a physiological infrastructure opposed to a psychic superstructure, but only levels of consciousness in the development of the human potential for connecting with the universe – the growth of the personality for the attainment of the highest ends of existence.

From the organic to the psychological, the physician comes across every human type and pathology in daily clinical practice, according to the emphasis in the patient's manifestations and the level of the vital problem. However, the foremost concern is to grasp the mental syndrome as the most faithful expression of the individual's constitution or vital unity.

In order to carry out a thorough case history to grasp the factors of personality and constitution, undetectable through laboratory tests or objective research, we must leave our closed, anti-psychological attitudes behind. Careful contact with the patient's emotional intimacy is more valuable than laboratory data.

It is increasingly difficult for mechanistic medicine to maintain that the mental and physical dysfunctions which underlie the pathological process are unrelated to the patient's moral disorder – that is, to the patient's values, expectations in life and attitude towards themselves as well as towards other human beings. To assist a patient without finding out about the circumstances in which they live and the psychological and spiritual substratum of their organic affection is clinically senseless. The patient's past, profession, attitude, emotional life and family environment give clues to the character and personality which have conditioned the pathological present. Thus, an individual diagnosis of the patient's disease through the symptoms of their psychological background is possible.

Pathological lesions and organic diseases are the products of a vital affection involving the whole person as they react to that continuous exchange between their motivating, conflicting internal forces and the external forces that mould them. Disease occurs when those internal and external forces are not in harmony.

The physician no longer asks what ails the patient, but who *is* the patient. This requires a detailed inquiry into the patient's somatic and structural condition, their nervous system, general symptoms and reactive modalities, and last but not least their feelings, dreams, desires, ambitions, current projects and needs. Nothing should be left in the dark, for it is precisely these life experiences that influence the person's biological equilibrium. Every psychic experience takes place within the organism, depending on it but actively influencing it at the same time. And if the goal of medicine is not to suppress symptoms but to cure the patient, the physician must attempt to understand the purposive meaning of such vital phenomena. Shaped not only by hereditary endowment but also by environmental factors, it is the patient's constitution that conditions both their resistance and their adaptation.

Still far from Pasteur's own requirements, constitutional pathology cannot yet offer a complete understanding of the underlying cause of disease. Hahnemann was able to explain the fundamental cause of disease in empirical terms, using the totality of symptoms gathered from pathogeneses,

In order to fulfil its true Hahnemannian purpose, homoeopathy must adhere to this anthropological quest, seeking to understand the patient as a biological unit in action. We should not even call homoeopathy psychosomatic, because the word still maintains the Cartesian concept of the body-mind split so dear to natural scientific medicine. Consciousness and will definitely influence the activity of the functional system.

However, a person's humour, drives, emotions, fatigue and over-valuation of ideas also depend on their functional system. There is indeed a reciprocal conditioning process: function determines the structure of the organ but, equally, function depends on structure.

Although the regulatory function of the autonomic nervous system is total and unitary, each organ and each function also has its own regulatory autonomy. In other words, each autonomic nervous function can, up to a certain limit, perform independently of the central diencephalic-hypophysial function that regulates the totality. Germs, a cellular product of the reticuloendothelial system, acquire their own capacity for infection. As represented by the ancient symbol of the serpent biting its tail, the entire autonomic system not only consists of the nerves that conduct stimuli, but also of hormones and cells which dynamically regulate the different functions in a unitary circle of interaction.

This explains why the practice of ameliorating symptoms with conventional (or even homoeopathic) prescriptions, whether for the purpose of draining or correcting an organic dysfunction, will have immediate results. Justified in irreversible cases, or when the reactive vitality has been exhausted, medications prescribed in this fashion act on the circumscribed pathogenic automatism of the localised complaint. However, partial improvements do not really cure; removing gallstones will not heal the liver patient. As long as medicine aspires only to improve and repair the functional or structural results of the true disease that involves the patient's whole life – made up of body, soul and spirit – it cannot go beyond the admittedly brilliant limits of a science concerned with physicochemical determinism, pathology and morphology. As long as medicine does not subordinate natural phenomena to the vital laws that go beyond physics, it will be unable to fulfil its essential mission – to truly cure the patient so that, acting from a level of freedom and self-decision, that person can attain the highest ends of their existence.

Simply to prescribe homoeopathic remedies does not confer the right to be a homoeopath. If the *Organon* is ignored, if one yields routinely to the localised concept of disease or systematically prescribes several remedies at one time, one is merely applying a symptomatic therapeutics with homoeopathic remedies. To understand symptoms means to encompass their retrospective history, in order to know their origin and subsequent evolution.

To those who state that this unicist or Hahnemannian homoeopathy is difficult to practise, we say yes – it is indeed no less difficult to practise than medicine itself. However, if the physician's training depends on the ability to be, and not only to know, then to be a homoeopath one must not only know but acquire the necessary faith. Only after having personally proved the remedial action of a remedy when correcting a chronic process, and only after having correctly interpreted and foreseen the meaning of this chronic process, can this faith be acquired. As Aristotle once declared: 'Plato is dear to me, but truth is dearer still.'

Chapter 15

The Practice of Homoeopathy II
(1962)

Personal experience in the practice of homoeopathy has confirmed my conviction that the physician cannot control the healing process until he has acquired a holistic clinical perspective of the patient, and perceived the radical unity of the morbid nucleus which must be cured. Without this perspective of each particular case, it is not possible to apply the simillimum that will stimulate the vital force towards cure. That is, the homoeopath must not be limited to the current symptom picture.

The success which homoeopathy clearly enjoys in the treatment of localised diseases with the similar remedy cannot be considered as any other than palliative measures, often leading to suppressions that are injurious to the patient's outcome. In this sense, homoeopathy is no less aggressive than conventional medicine or any other therapeutic system. To suppress organic or localised processes, while neglecting their derivative function, is to lose sight of the nucleus of the chronic affection. The disease may be suppressed but the patient slips away. No matter how careful the prescription based on general modalities, we cannot find all the characteristic symptoms that allow for individualisation of the constitutional simillimum in the current disease. Furthermore, the remedy that covers the general modalities of the current moment may also reveal old latent symptoms, allowing us to diagnose the simillimum that reflects a previous stage, and in this manner arrive at the constitutional remedy from childhood.

Clinical observations have verified that the diseases which occur in a patient's life are not isolated episodes. They are successive aspects of the same diathetic state that may emerge from a latent state, due to a specific harmful stimulus of microbial, traumatic, dietary, climatic or emotional origin. It is not a question of 'wanting' an illness, but of having the potential to harbour it. Only those who are susceptible to certain physical or emotional impacts may fall ill in certain ways.

The series of acute episodes which a patient may have suffered throughout his life are strictly conditioned by that person's individual terrain.

The Hahnemannian concept of latent psora – which coincides with the concept of diathesis, or constitutional disposition – does not refer to the remnant of acute infections or to certain deficiency or metabolic states. It relates to a permanent dynamic disturbance which compromises the very core of vital activity – and it is there that anxiety, an essential symptom of psora, is the first morbid substratum that a person experiences.

Before any infection occurs, the vital disturbance which predisposed the patient to the disease already existed, increasing the patient's anxiety and stress levels.

The surgeon can verify that he has removed a cancerous stomach. However, he cannot claim that the patient has been cured of the primary anxiety that led to the ulcer which preceded the final cancer.

The homoeopathic perspective of chronic disease enables the physician to enhance the healing mechanism at deeper levels and to deal with the current disease as a direct continuation of previous diseases. Even though the type of relationship between the final cancer and the preceding gastric anxiety may not be understood, the homoeopath may still claim to know the face of cancer as it could never be known in the laboratory.

It is not in the virus but in the human mind that the factors which determine the cancerous disease, or the characteristic elements of that disturbance of the vital energy which condition the physiology and pathological structure of the organism, are to be found.

But if that research into the patient's mentality is to have any real clinical value, the homoeopath must first draw up a complete life history, including any moral, hygienic or drug-related transgressions that the patient has committed and decide whether the case is suitable for homoeopathic treatment or not, and whether it is curable or incurable.

The greatest loss of prestige to homoeopathy is due to a bad choice of cases and an incorrect application of remedies.

One German patient, a 32-year-old mother of four, had suffered from a chronic pansinusitis for the previous two years. She had undergone many treatments, all to no avail. Before undergoing surgery, she turned to homoeopathy. She had a suppurating rhinitis and felt a constant burning pain in her sinuses and maxillaries.

This patient's clinical history revealed that she had also suffered from gastrointestinal ailments with pains in the right hypochondrium and epigastrium after eating, much belching and flatulence, a sensation as if she had a stone in the pit of her stomach, an apprehensive reverberation in the stomach brought on by the slightest cause for anxiety, and pasty, frothy and offensive stools.

Upon asking about her mental state, I met with some resistance on her part. She claimed to have turned to homoeopathy in order to avoid having her paranasal sinuses removed, just as the person who had recommended homoeopathy to her had thereby avoided having hers removed. I explained that her acquaintance had also been thoroughly examined and that it was not just a matter of curing her sinusitis but of curing her in her entirety, and that I therefore needed to know her life history. She told me that ever since her first menstruation she had been afflicted with nervous disorders, and that these had worsened progressively until her marriage. Later on, her husband, a wealthy man, and the physicians she consulted advised her to see a psychiatrist.

Eleven years before her current sinusitis, immediately after the birth of her first child, her condition was aggravated with attacks of irritability and anger, alternating with depression. She had had odd sensations that made her feel very insecure. For example, she felt as if she were double and disintegrated, with her body and mind separate from each other. She also felt as if her body were very fragile and could dissolve or break at the slightest physical or psychological impact.

She had fits of anger and intense exasperation, as well as depression and phobic and obsessive ideas. She was treated with several sedatives and was interned in a psychiatric clinic, finally undergoing hypnosis and electroshock treatment. Because she continued in the same state, which finally led to a manic-depressive symptom picture, she was again interned in a clinic where, after a thorough medical examination, she was prescribed sedatives and hypnotic therapy, followed by psychoanalysis.

This woman's hypomanic crises and deep melancholic depressions improved, but her obsessive ideas did not abandon her for a single moment. She returned to Buenos Aires, where she continued with her psychotherapy as well as treatment for her nerves until, two years before consulting me a violent, acute coryza with fever appeared, as well as a general breakdown which subsided five days after being treated with antibiotics. From that moment on, while her fits of anger, melancholy and depressions improved, she developed a purulent rhinitis in her paranasal cavities that was resistant to antibiotics and vaccine therapy. At that point, while her mental symptom picture was being treated with psychotherapy, her sinus condition was being treated separately as a localised illness. Undoubtedly, her nasal and paranasal ailment was vicariously fulfilling certain mental functions and yet her mental problems and physical condition were being treated as two different diseases.

Even though the physician cannot perform a scientific experiment to establish a correspondence between pathological change and what transpires in the psyche, one cannot dispute the fact that mental symptoms certainly do have clinically discernible correlations with physiological processes.

This woman's localised symptoms had improved her mental state somewhat, but she still suffered from ideas, sensations and other general symptoms. She had the sensation of perceiving things as if from somewhere outside her body. She reported 'feeling divided', as if she were split in two, and not knowing who she was.

She also had the sensation of acting and thinking incorrectly. She was tormented by fixed ideas that she could not control and which were relieved only when she was with her psychotherapist and felt protected. Only then was her sense of guilt assuaged – even though she did not know what it was that she had done wrong. She would pray to God to forgive her for her bad thoughts, even though she did not know what they were. To escape this mental confusion, she constantly thought of suicide.

Because she felt her body to be so fragile, she did not want to be touched. She even asked her husband and children not to come too near her because she felt they could harm her with the slightest contact.

Nothing satisfied or interested her. Dull and unable to concentrate, she could not read and with such sadness and aversion to life, she wished for death to escape from her tedium.

She felt a sensation of apprehension in the pit of her stomach as if a stone was there which prevented her from eating. At 54kg and 1.63 metres tall, she was also very thin and anaemic.

In general, she was worse during wet and cold weather. She had rhinitis with a copious, purulent, non-excoriating discharge. Her menses were abundant, prolonged and frequent, sometimes having two menstrual periods in a single month. Her symptoms, then, were the following:

Anxiety of conscience (as if guilty of a crime)
Confusion as to her identity
Delusion of being double
Aversion to being touched

Loathing of life
Discontented
Stupefaction of mind
Apprehension in stomach
Worse from wet weather
Coryza with copious discharge
Menses, copious

As a small child, she had had measles and diphtheria. Her tonsils had been removed at the age of nine; her appendix at eighteen. At the time of the first consultation, she had four children and had been treated several times by her gynaecologist, who cauterised her cervix to suppress the abundant, fetid and excoriating discharge she had had until two years previously.

Her father had died of stomach cancer and her mother was diabetic. She was an only child.

Because of her confused identity, guilt feelings and obsessive character with manic-depressive tendencies, it was clear that this patient was dynamically deranged due to a sycotic background.

Reference to the materia medica, verified by the repertory, led to Thuja – a diagnosis which was not based on her localised process but on her mental symptoms. I prescribed three doses in the 12c, 30c and 200c potencies, each to be taken at twelve-hourly intervals.

The morning after her dose of Thuja 200c she woke up feeling irritable and confused, which reminded her of her worst attacks in the past. She had dreamt of her mother – whom she had hated since she was a very young child – especially after the death of her father to whom she was emotionally attached. She wept bittterly, feeling regretful and guilty for this uncontrollable feeling.

Five days later she began to suppurate copiously through the nose and the orifice where an upper molar had been extracted seven months before.

This aggravation lasted a week, during which she could not sleep. Her sinuses, nose and mouth suppurated copiously; she had much mental confusion and lost 3kg, which intensified her general weakness and made her sink into a deplorable physical condition. However, after eight to ten days she began to feel calmer and more self-confident. Her pain and general malaise subsided and she began to eat with a good appetite, gained weight and strength and, above all, no longer felt as if her body were separate from her mind – the sensation which had accompanied her for years.

Two months later her mental condition had changed completely. She no longer had obsessive ideas, depressions, sadness or aversion to life. Neither did she feel as if her body were fragile, and therefore for the first time could enjoy her children's hugs and kisses.

Although attenuated, the suppuration still continued through her nose, having stopped through her mouth. Five months later, she gained 8kg, had acute periodical attacks of coryza with a discrete discharge of pus, and her obsessive mental state had disappeared. However, she still hated her mother even though she felt guilty about it.

In the course of two years after this aggravation, she took two doses of Thuja, one at 10M and one at 50M, which finally cured her neurosis and sinusitis, thus saving her from shock therapy and surgery. If it had not been for homoeopathy, it is unlikely that she would have recovered.

Another patient, a 37-year-old widow, came to my office because she had been told she had a cyst in her right ovary which needed to be operated on.

Four years earlier she had had another cyst removed from her left ovary and, eight months after that, was operated on again because a new cyst supposedly had grown in the same place. (It turned out that this was really one and a half metres of gauze which had been left there during her first operation.)

After this experience she understandably wished to avoid surgery at all costs and therefore turned to homoeopathy.

As a child this woman was thin and emaciated and had always had poor health. She had had measles, whooping cough, frequent attacks of bronchitis and suppurating otitis in both ears, having undergone tapping in order to drain off the fluid. She had a chronic catarrh of the naso-pharynx during the whole of her childhood, periodically aggravated by strong acute attacks of bronchitis, until at sixteen she contracted pleurisy on her right side with serofibrinous fluid. At the age of twenty she married a sickly man who died ten months later of a heart attack.

Still thin, she had frequent colds, pains in her pulmonary bases, and no matter how well she ate, could not gain weight. After her marriage she had started to have a copious, mucous and bloody leucorrhoea which was locally treated and suppressed.

At the age of twenty-nine corticopleuritis was diagnosed, from which she slowly recovered with strong antibiotics. After her bout of corti-copleuritis, her vaginal discharge reappeared and one and a half years later, after receiving ineffective treatments, an ovarian cyst was diagnosed. This was removed four years before she first consulted me.

Her father had been asthmatic and died of cancer of the mediastinum.

At the time of her first interview, this woman's mental symptom picture was the following:

Much nervous debility, hypersensitive, irritable.

Physically and mentally tired, everything accomplished with a great effort; even coming to meals an enormous strain.

Full of doubts, deciding on the most trivial matters a terrible agony.

Nothing satisfied her. Very changeable, she wanted one thing after another. Never sticking to anything, she had a constant desire to travel and change her surroundings or occupation. Uncertain of everything, she constantly changed physicians.

Afraid of dying if left alone, and always sought companionship.

Physically and mentally restless, with an overwhelming desire to be busy at something new and different.

Her physical symptoms were the following:

Frequent coryzas; a tendency to take cold easily, even upon entering a cold room or stepping into a cold place.

In spite of her extreme sensitivity to cold, a need to breathe open, fresh air.

Emaciated state in spite of her good appetite and adequate diet.

I prescribed Tuberculinum 1M, which covered the totality of her symptoms. She gained four kilograms and, eight months later, her gynaecologist found that her cyst had diminished considerably and advised her to continue with her homoeopathic treatment.

Two years later the cyst had disappeared completely, but her nervousness, irritability and restlessness persisted, along with a profuse perspiration at dawn and a marked sensitivity to cold. Since Tuberculinum was no longer acting, I prescribed Silica 1M, albeit without much conviction because her symptom picture was so vague. However, a year and a half later she had a well-defined symptom picture, made up of the following symptoms:

An accentuated return of sadness, melancholy and apprehension with anxiety concerning her future, and a marked tendency towards weeping.

Great fear of people, whom she avoided, and aversion towards members of her family, as well as certain people with whom she terminated her friendship.

Very sensitive to music, which provoked weeping and anguish.

She empathised excessively with animals, to the point of weeping when she saw a small animal ill.

Copious catarrh of the nasopharynx.
Scanty menses with amenorrhoea of 1-2 months. Constantly felt as if
her menses were about to appear.

After repertorisation, her syndrome was the following:

Aversion to certain persons
Aversion to members of family
Fear of people
Sensitive to music
Sympathetic
Catarrh, postnasal
Menses, scanty

Natrum Carbonicum 1M and Natrum Carbonicum 10M brought this
patient back to normal. Today, she has completely recovered, weighs
65kg, has no colds or fatigue even though she works hard, and has a
happy and calm disposition.

Her ovarian cyst, which was to have been surgically removed, did not
reappear. Thus this patient's general state, emotions and mental symptoms corresponded first to Tuberculinum's symptom picture, and afterwards to that of Natrum Carbonicum.

It is a patient's mental and emotional symptoms which decide a
prescription, as long as they agree with general symptoms that refer to
temperature, climate, movement, food likes and dislikes and other
factors. The keynote symptom must be backed up by general symptoms,
mainly by reactions to weather changes. However, even after a detailed
repertorisation, the determining symptom of the good simillimum is
always mental.

As a scientist, the homoeopath carefully analyses and scrutinises the
patient's symptoms. Then, as an artist, he must discover the patient's
true character behind the defences.

Repertorisation will always yield two or three remedies which are
similar in the general modalities, but which oppose each other in the
mental aspect and which, because they are similar, antidote each other.

For example, one woman's repertorisation pointed equally to Sepia
and to Pulsatilla. At first, given her affable and docile nature, I was
inclined towards Pulsatilla. Later on, upon discovering that she was
dissatisfied in her home, that she sent her two-year-old son to kindergarten and her six-year-old son to an all-day school and remained alone
with her husband, towards whom she felt aversion, I diagnosed Sepia.

Because of her good breeding and manners, Sepia's characteristic
symptoms of indifference towards her children and aversion towards

her husband had been eclipsed by an apparently agreeable and sub-missive attitude. During her second visit, her husband revealed another mental symptom which corroborated my diagnosis: aversion towards the physician as well as the treatment, which also belongs to Sepia. The results were optimal and, therapeutically speaking, we won her trust.

One man had a symptom picture of emaciation, mucous and bloody diarrhoea, intense thirst, craving for salt, a tendency to take cold, fear of misfortune and insanity. These symptoms are shared by Natrum Muriaticum and Phosphorus. He also had restlessness, which can be confused with hurry.

When active, this man was nevertheless physically weak and lacking in willpower. He enthusiastically started projects but never finished them, soon passing on to other things. Phosphorus behaves in this way. On the other hand, Natrum Muriaticum has more hurry than restless-ness and never starts a task without completing it, albeit carrying it out with haste. Phosphorus was therefore the remedy in this case.

One woman, whose chronic headaches improved with Sepia, pre-scribed for indifference in her affections and aversion towards her children, suddenly, five months after her last dose of Sepia 10M, reported that she did not have any more headaches, that she felt well and happier, and had normal relationships. However, she felt a great apprehension when driving her car, fearing an accident. Even when her husband drove she felt very disturbed in the middle of traffic, and had even considered moving to a suburb in order to avoid it. But when I enquired more deeply into all the sensations she felt, she said she was embarrassed that she also felt a great aversion to public places, because she could not tolerate the dirty smell of people in crowds, and that precisely this, together with the aversion to being in a heated room, made her think she could not be psychologically normal.

It is easy to see that the four symptoms:

Worse on riding
Worse from unpleasant odours
Worse in warm room
Fear of insanity

led to Sulphur, which completed the cure in this patient with her chronic headaches and a difficult marriage situation, due to psychological conflicts derived from her morbid state.

One 64-year-old man who looked well stopped by my office just to greet me. He had last been my patient twenty years previously and since then had not needed to consult any doctor whatsoever.

Looking in his file, I found that two years before his last visit he had come to my office complaining of a duodenal ulcer, confirmed by X-ray, for which he had been advised to undergo surgery. His localised symptoms had been heartburn and an excessive production of hyperchloric acid in the stomach. He had to take food every two hours, and when he took dairy products he was temporarily relieved of the burning pains in his stomach. He had also had rheumatic pains in the larger joints, headaches, constipation and haemorrhoids. His general symptoms had been: hot; sensation of heat on the soles of the feet; rheumatic pains worse by dry, cold weather and better by damp weather; intense thirst; craving for ice-cold drinks, salt and sweets. His mental symptoms included fear of the dark and of death.

I had prescribed one dose of Medorrhinum 200c and then a placebo. The man had saved the old slips for the subsequent prescriptions I had filled out and even brought them that day for me to see: another placebo two months after the first one, then one dose of Medorrhinum 10M a month later, and finally Medorrhinum CM the day of his last visit.

He reported that his cure had been rapid and definitive. A few months after his last dose of Medorrhinum CM he had had a bout of shingles in the left thoracic base. But he did not consult me, he said, because he had remembered my admonitions that any releases through mucus or skin had to be respected and not suppressed. Ever since then he had enjoyed perfect health, merely by clean living in every sense. He never had a stomach symptom again.

This prescription, filled out many years ago, based on fear of the dark, fear of death, better by wet weather, craving for salt and sweets, burning sensation on the soles of the feet and craving for cold drinks, decided the cure of a patient otherwise destined for the operating table.

The single remedy, prescribed on the basis of the patient's general and mental characteristics, together with the physician's firm and expectant attitude regarding any new and old symptoms which may appear in the course of a treatment, are the best guarantees of a sure success in homoeopathy's highest aim: to cure the patient.

Chapter 16

Child Psychology in Homoeopathy
(1963)

In homoeopathy, child psychology is studied as a symptomatic expression of diathesis. Character and behaviour faithfully reflect the morbid temperament which, in turn, responds both to the child's unique constitutional susceptibility and to emotional stimuli from the child's environment.

By matching the child's behavioural symptoms and reactions with the major remedies of the materia medica, homoeopathy can improve the constitution. Speculative psychology has no place in homoeopathy except to help us confirm the validity of mental symptoms. From Freud to the present time, most schools of psychoanalysis acknowledge that the constitutional predisposition is an important factor in childhood behavioural disorders.

In his theory of chronic diseases, Hahnemann inductively concluded that psora, a dynamic derangement of vital equilibrium, expresses itself mainly through anxiety. Psora, then, is that primal state of susceptibility, irritability or homoeostatic imbalance which conditions the terrain for infection. From psora springs the basic existential anxiety which every child brings into the world, expressed as primal withdrawal and fear of life upon separation from the mother.

To experience anxiety is to long for something, to anticipate with fear something that will relieve a tension caused by an unsatisfied need, such as the sensation of hunger – the original expression of our instinct for self-preservation.

For Hahnemann, symptoms pertaining to the unconscious will – what psychoanalysts call the libido – determine the patient's characteristic symptom picture. This is so because the underlying derangement of the psoric miasm is grounded in the instinct for self-preservation, and its natural outlet is the digestive system. Disorders of the appetite, food likes and dislikes, the compulsive need for salt, sugar, fat, calcium, stimulants or indigestible foods, which are part of homoeopathic symptomatology, as well as psychological keynotes such as

117

anticipation, apprehension, epileptic aura, and other symptoms localised in the stomach, indicate that the digestive system reflects the primal tension caused by the instinctive need for self-preservation. This is deeply experienced by the child as a vague anxiety or a confused fear of annihilation.

Psora is not an infectious state, nor a toxic residue from previous infections, nor a disturbance created by a deficiency. Underlying all pathology, psora is a state of hypersensitivity or allergic susceptibility. Psora is a dynamic alarm signal for our internal imbalance, produced by our instinctive conflict of self-preservation. And we say 'instinctive conflict' because, opposed to this basic core of anxiety that conditions the ancestral fear of death is the life instinct – the vital force which moves the child to react with rage and aggression in order to neutralise the intolerable, corroding sensation of hunger. Because the outer world does not yet exist for the child, and because the child cannot bear to be separated from its mother, he or she projects this unbearable sensation on to the mother, and with it the aggression necessary for neutralising it.

The infant will bite the mother's breast that gives it sustenance. Later on, the child may even hit her, and later still will develop many forms of aggression against the world, experienced as a surrogate mother. During his lifetime the child will struggle with this conflict between anxiety and aggression, representing the opposite and interacting forces that animate all human beings and which are present in all physical, chemical, biological and psychological processes: attraction and repulsion, anabolism and catabolism, creation and destruction, love and hate.

The process of growth, and thereby of healing, in the child consists in severing the umbilical cord that unites him with the mother, thus resolving the conflict between anxiety and aggression. While anxiety ties the child to the mother, father or any other person (later on it may even be spouse and children), aggression creates guilt feelings which lead to the obsessive symptom pictures that afflict so many human beings.

The subtle, insidious and varied ways in which the child's precarious defence mechanisms respond to this basic conflict between anxiety and aggression are still a puzzle for psychology. As can be gleaned from every child's symptom picture, these defence mechanisms involve insecurity, uncertainty and instability. And although a person's psychic mechanism can be influenced to a certain extent from the course, clinical reasoning and conjecture can never penetrate the nature of the deep experience which gives rise to it. As Saint Augustine said, 'What then is time? I know what it is if no one asks me what it is; but if I want to explain it to someone who has asked me, I find that I do not know.'

Thus, the child defends itself from this basic conflict between anxiety and aggression by reacting with organic disease and with various forms of behaviour, according to their unique functional stigmatisation. The highly potentised homoeopathic remedy which strikes that psoric core of anxiety is the only recourse available to medicine for influencing the patient's dynamic constitutional plane from which that basic conflict springs.

I saw a girl who had suffered a sprain in her right foot ten months before. Fifteen days after the incident her right knee had swollen with much pain. The fluid was tapped and drained, she wore a cast and was treated for rheumatism. (The guinea-pig test was negative.) She was given twenty-five bottles of streptomycin as well as cortisone and other drugs until, as a last resort, exploratory surgery was suggested. Except for a bout of measles at the age of three, this young patient's pathological history was almost nil. However, her emotional symptom picture was quite clear. As a very small child she feared being alone and would often tremble with terror when night approached. She constantly expressed her anguished fear of the possibility of losing her mother or her father, who both pampered her and to whom she was very much attached.

She also woke from nightmares crying, and as she grew older her family observed that she developed a fear of physical weakness and of not being as 'as clever as the other girls', as she put it. On the whole, she was physically healthy and was developing normally until, a year before coming to see me, her father had died of a heart attack. She then suffered an emotional collapse with a loss of consciousness, followed by inconsolable weeping. Three weeks after her father's death she went to the cemetery, and near his tomb she sprained her foot. Two weeks later her knee swelled up and a month after that she had a serious infection in a molar which turned into an abscess, followed by influenza with pulmonary congestion and, a few weeks later, suppurating conjunctivitis in both eyes.

The connection between this chain of ailments and the emotional shock of her father's death (both father and mother are a single person in a child's emotional life) was so obvious that there was no room for doubt in my mind, or in her family's mind as well.

This young patient's latent psora had been unleashed by emotional factors. Previously hidden under an apparent state of equilibrium, her constitutional symptom picture was now revealed. Pathologically oriented medicine does not make sense of morbid phenomena such as these and studies them as unrelated episodes.

By contrast, homoeopathy, without speculating on the mechanism that corresponds to the somatisation of anxiety, verifies the patient's underlying mental state as expressed through pathology. This girl's general physical and psychological symptom picture was the following:

Before her trouble with her knee, she had had the following symptoms:

Fear that something would happen to her or her family (which did in fact come to pass with her father's death)

Fear of the night and of being alone

Fear of weakness and disease

Fear of not being as capable as other girls (in other words, fear of psychological imbalance or feeble-mindedness)

Apprehension in the stomach, as if something would rise from the stomach to the head

Sensation of levitating

Cold sensation in certain parts of the body: head, abdomen, her bad knee

Cold feet with cold sweat; sometimes, a fleeting sensation of internal heat

As a very small child, profuse perspiration of the head, soaking her pillow

There was no doubt at all that this was a Calcarea Carbonica symptom picture. Indeed, a single dose of Calcarea Carbonica 1M brought about a radical change in this young patient, not only solving her knee problem – which healed completely, the swelling having disappeared and her mobility restored – but promoting a general recovery, especially concerning her mental symptoms. Having freed her conscience from the need to inflict self-punishment for the loss of her father, she went through a normal mourning process and later recovered her joy in living. A few months later, after more doses of Calcarea Carbonica, she enjoyed a psychological state that she had never had before, free from fears and terrors, and with a boost in her mental ability.

This was five years ago and today her knee is completely cured. And this cure was brought about by diagnosing her mental and not her localised symptoms.

Years before current trends in psychosomatic thought, which attempt to understand the patient's clinical reality as an indivisible body-mind unit, Hahnemann had stated that bodily diseases are not distinct from mental diseases. He maintained that even though the mind sometimes appropriates physical suffering, there are always bodily symptoms in a psychopathological disorder and there are always psychological alterations in an organic disease. Dynamism cannot be separated from structure. However, it is the soul which rules over the body, just as the spirit directs the soul, so that, for the homoeopath, the emotional symptoms which structure the personality and character are also those which determine the modalities which express the child's constitution. If the homoeopath attentively observes the child's psychic reactions, he will be able to find the simillimum which will correct both body and mind.

A four-year-old girl was brought to my office with a subacute oedema in both knees and ankles. Her joints were painful in several points and she had great difficulty in walking. Her general condition was deficient; thin, pale and very nervous. She cried easily and suffered from frequent headaches with vomiting.

The previous year she had had her first attack of acute rheumatic fever, reflecting Bouillaud's symptom picture. Her joints being very much affected, she was in bed for seventy days. After heavy doses of antibiotics, vitamins and analgesics, she pulled through her acute state only to become a chronic patient, her morbid affection still being unresolved.

All resources were exhausted, including a tonsillectomy six months before coming to see me, with no improvement. She was very irritable, in addition to the pains in her joints, nightly fever, headaches, vomiting, constipation, extreme emaciation and sensitivity to cold. She also had frequent attacks of rage, strong nervous reactions at the slightest contradiction, followed by trembling and a state of exhaustion which made her sink into a deep, almost stuporous sleep.

With the fever she was anxious, restless and very talkative. Always capricious, nothing satisfied her. She would ask for food which she rejected after barely tasting it; she whined and complained constantly. One revealing symptom that belongs to tubercular symptom pictures was that she could not bear to see anything white or light reflected on white surfaces, to the point that her mother had to cover the mirrors in the house.

This mental symptom picture characterised by irritability, instability, loquacity when feverish and an intolerance of white surfaces, together with the worsening of her pains in wet weather, headaches with weeping and emaciation, led to Tuberculinum Koch 200c.

Although this case reflected Tuberculinum's mental symptom picture, I could nevertheless not find a single, well-defined, particular psychological trait. As usually happens when the tubercular miasm is awakened in infancy, children suddenly become very irritable. They may throw temper tantrums followed by trembling, weakness and exhaustion. They become restless and capricious, with a desire to change whatever activity they are doing. They constantly feel the desire to do something different, although they do not know what it may be. As they grow older, they do not know what to study or what to do with their lives. They wish to travel, change their environment and occupation. They are extremely sensitive to light, music, noise, pain and all sensory impressions.

Even when nosodes such as Tuberculinum are applied by strictly matching their images to the patient's symptoms, they cannot remove the dynamic morbid substratum which, at its deepest levels, constitutionally conditions the patient. Only the antipsoric mineral which strikes the cell's dyscrasic ion can cure the underlying psora. Produced from normal or pathological substances, nosodes usually do not cure psora, but they do cause the patient's constitutional symptom picture to surface, which will then enable the physician to find the simillimum. This is precisely what I expected and obtained with this young patient.

One month after the dose of Tuberculinum Koch 200c she was much better, was eating and resting well, had gained weight and was free of pain. Her joints were no longer swollen and her character was much improved. She did not need another dose of the remedy until ten months later, when she developed an acute laryngotracheal catarrh as well as a recurrence of pains in her knees and ankles, but without the oedema as before.

During those ten months, I had seen the child five times and had prescribed only a placebo in order to appease her mother, who could not believe that a cure had been brought about by a single dose. Nevertheless, four or five months before her next visit, her parents reported a striking change in their daughter's behaviour.

During one particular thunderstorm, she had become very frightened. When this happened again, her family noticed that she was terrified and very excitable while the thunderstorm was gathering, but that once it started raining she collapsed from exhaustion, and slept deeply.

After this fright she became very restless, starting at every sound. She developed a fear of burglars and darkness and did not want to be left alone for a single moment. Also, her family was astonished to discover that she now had a tendency to be obsessively concerned about other people's welfare – perhaps as a consequence of her marked desire for pampering and consolation. In contrast to her previous character, she now felt sorry for any person or animal. If family members happened to be ill, she wanted to take their meals to them. She constantly asked what she could do to help other people and showed genuine concern and fear for what could happen to her family, especially to her grandmother, whom she loved very much.

Together with her fear of burglars and the dark, her jumpiness and restlessness, there was no doubt that the symptom 'Sympathetic', so clearly defined, had now surfaced as a psychological characteristic after this fright with the thunderstorm. Sympathy was so marked that it was now this young patient's determinative symptom, which clearly indicated Phosphorus.

After one dose of Phosphorus 200c she never suffered from pain again. Her rheumatism was completely cured and her general condition improved enormously. She gained weight, had a good appetite and slept well. Unlike Natrum Muriaticum, who rejects sympathy, she was still fond of being pampered, which is typical of Phosphorus. Not only do Phosphorus children crave sympathy, consolation and petting, they are also very affectionate themselves and love to bestow their kisses on everyone.

Phosphorus was the simillimum in this case, which had nevertheless been latent, hidden under a Tuberculinum picture. As happens with the correctly prescribed nosode, Tuberculinum roused this young patient's true constitutional symptom picture.

Perhaps some day medicine will be able to devise the formula for the psychosomatic relationship between specific conflicts or psychological complexes and specific organic functions. Nevertheless, clinical experience shows that when the homoeopath painstakingly deals with the child's mental problem according to the general physical reactions, he is able to modify that child's unique disposition to disease and neurosis. Mental symptoms are always the indisputable basis of homoeopathic prescription.

One six-year-old girl was brought by her mother for a condylomatous wart the size of a pea on her upper left eyelid. This child also suffered from vulvitis with mucous leucorrhoea. She also had enuresis, pains in the joints of her knees and ankles, anorexia; she was sensitive to cold, although this last symptom was not clearly defined.

This blatantly sycotic symptom picture could easily make one think of Thuja. However, her mother volunteered that her child's character had changed before the wart appeared. She had developed an intense fear of the dark, was afraid of being left alone, could not sleep with the lights out and obsessively ensured that all the doors were locked at night. This mental syndrome, also sycotic, led to Causticum. Eight days after a single dose of Causticum 200c her wart fell off and her nightly terrors, enuresis and the pains in her joints disappeared.

How can we explain the relationship between anxiety and a wart? What is the specific connection between a psychodynamic factor such as fear of the dark and a pathological phenomenon such as abnormal tissue growth? Do psychodynamic factors determine pathological phenomena?

With our limited concepts of physiological chemistry this has no explanation, which is why these concerns are generally absent from clinical practice. But when we think in terms of dynamics, such connections make sense. The sycotic miasm is a deranged exacerbation of the physiological function of reproduction. This is why the cell proliferates in a disorderly fashion, producing warts, condylomata, tumours and all kinds of abnormal tissue growths. This activation springs from the same vital stimulus which, biologically, makes the cell reproduce; psychically, it is transformed into instinct. It is not surprising, then, that this girl developed fear, anxiety and an obsessive neurosis when faced with the sycotic exacerbation of her aggressive erotic instinct – which she projected as a threat and from which she defended herself with locked doors and burning lightbulbs.

The constitutional homoeopathic remedy may well be the biological solution which Freud cried out for in the difficult course of psychoanalytic treatment.

As in every human being, the child's underlying problem is that of freeing the vital force, the *vis medicatrix*, from the conflicts roused by psoric anxiety and aggression, both of which hamper psychological growth. As we have seen, the law of cure applies not only to the process of centrifugal release but also to the dynamic evolution of the psyche – from the childish conflict between anxiety and aggression to the psychological maturity to a freely giving and loving attitude.

At the end of her treatment, one 18-year-old girl clearly and spontaneously expressed this psychological transformation in herself. She had been a sad, melancholy child, poor in spirit, anxious and agitated, who would wake in anguish and who suffered from much irritability and destructive fury. She was very sensitive to noise and could not bear to be spoken to in a loud tone, nor to be touched. Although she was very intelligent and imaginative she could not apply herself to her studies, because she was incapable of prolonged mental effort.

Her pale, emaciated appearance, her anxious character and her attacks of rage caused her parents to bring her to my office. They told me that ever since she was a small child she had developed an obsessive, guilt-ridden character, as if she had made some mistake or done something bad. She worked in a kindergarten and confessed that she was afraid of harming the children, in spite of being very fond of them and wanting to take care of them. She felt anxiety at the slightest separation from her mother and panicked at the thought of losing her. She constantly felt a kind of anxiety or fear as if life required something of her, although she was unable to discern what it was. This feeling would surface when faced with any circumstance in which she had to see someone or fulfil a previous commitment.

Her symptom picture was made up as follows:

Anxiety of conscience
Nervous anticipation
Obsessive character
Sensitive to noise
Headaches, better by rubbing head vigorously
Worse by cold and wet weather
Frequent colds
Profuse perspiration at dawn
Foot sweat
Chronic constipation
Chronic blepharitis with recurrent styes

Her constitutional remedy was Silica. I prescribed three doses: first, Silica 200c, Silica 1M two months later, and another dose of Silica 1M four months later.

Six months after the last dose of Silica her general condition was much improved: her tiredness had disappeared, she had gained weight and even her fingernails were stronger. Aside from her general physical improvement, I quote her own words regarding her mental and emotional state:

When I look back I now realise how much my attitude towards life has changed. I was consumed by a terrible fear of losing my mother and constantly demanded that everything be given to me: affection, help, moral support, protection for my loved ones. I had an insatiable need for reassurance, which never calmed my anxiety. Today, I feel capable of giving, of helping, of doing something for somebody, of taking care of my mother, of living for purposes other than concern for myself. Life has taken on a new meaning, because I now feel that I have cured my selfishness and no longer worry only about myself; in short, I believe that only recently have I grown up and become a real person. When I came to see you I was undergoing psycho-analysis, which I left shortly afterwards because I didn't need it any more. I leaned on my analyst for support, but I felt a sense of freedom growing in me which I had never known before. Then I left him for good as my fears of losing my loved ones dropped away.

These thoughts which she shared eloquently with me describe the emotional transformation that she underwent under the influence of her constitutional remedy. I must mention that leaving her psychoanalyst did not cause her to transfer her dependency on to me, because she visited me only six times in the course of almost two years. As this patient reported, she had attained psychological maturity, getting over the childhood mechanism of dependency which was detrimental to her development. This is what the homoeopathic remedy can do, when it stimulates the vital impulse towards growth and cure from the deepest biological level of the will from where the child goes through the painful process of growth.

When based on a detailed analysis of mental and physical symptoms, homoeopathy can solve a child's psychological problems. When correctly prescribed, the homoeopathic remedy can touch the con-stitutional core, making it possible to metabolise the primary psoric anxiety which, with sycotic eroticism and syphilitic aggression, together create the child's elaborate neurotic defence mechanisms which are so difficult to treat in psychotherapy.

Chapter 17

Homoeopathic Clinical Practice
(1964)

CASE 6

Mr M.B., age 49, has suffered from diabetes for eleven years. In his own words:

'I functioned almost normally with insulin for a while; but five years ago I developed an ulcer on the sole of one foot, which wouldn't heal for a long time; eventually it did heal but another ulcer developed on my other foot and I was beginning to develop gangrene. However, Dr Detinis saved my foot without surgery.

Two or three months ago I started feeling a pain in my heart and liver. This pain rises, becomes stronger and bothers me. It makes me think I have a bad heart. Anything I do, even walking, brings on the pain. I have resigned myself to dying. I'm not afraid of these things. I resign myself – I am a theosophist, so I've learned not to fear death. I believe that life is nothing but a learning field, and that life or being is eternal and manifests itself in different bodies. I am resigned. I am not interested in prolonging my life more than necessary. I am very nervous, terribly nervous. I have abandoned everything that used to interest me, such as philosophy and theosophy, because I believe my life is over. I am also a freemason. I used to profess all these things with a great interest, but now I am not interested in going to meetings any more; sometimes I attend them, but as soon as I'm there, I want to leave and be by myself. The same thing happens at home; everyone is happy watching TV or doing something else, but I go to my room and lie down. I experience this solitude, which makes me nervous, and start to feel that pain I mentioned. The pain rises and I have to inhale alcohol or take a pill for it.

I always had normal blood pressure, but lately I have 200 or 210, a lot higher than before. When I take the medicine the pain goes away, but if I feel nervous it comes back, and I can't work or walk. I am taking 40 units of insulin every morning. I also have a slight mechanical problem: I need to have a piece of bone removed which bothers me. But what bothers me the most is that I feel that my life is over. I am saying goodbye to people. I have no fear because I believe that death is only a stage. I like to be alone, read, organise lectures on theosophy, and mentally I lecture alone, but when the time comes to deliver them in public, I don't show up.

Right now I feel nervous and I'm starting to feel that pain again. If this sensation would only pass I would feel all right; when I don't feel pain I'm another person, much more communicative. Generally, I avoid people. I'm also troubled by other things. I'm married. If I want to make love I can't, because the pain starts again. As soon as I think of making love, it starts. Instead of giving me pleasure, it depresses me, makes me ill.

My only consolation is that mentally I feel fine; I read and I can assimilate what I read. I can give talks on topics I know about without using notes. I like to sit down and say what comes to mind. The same thing occurs with my painting. For instance, if I see some still life, I observe it carefully and then I paint it without looking at it. I try to paint what the scene means to me, not just copy it. Many people don't understand me. I try to interpret rather than just copy. If several artists were to paint the same scene, in the end the only different one would be mine. If one wants to copy something, one might as well take a photograph. On the canvas, I paint what the tree means to me; so the uninitiated don't understand me. All my problems are like this.

I feel at my worst at night time. I sleep for about fifteen minutes and then I wake up with that pain. This happens before midnight and I sit up in bed until 3 or 4 a.m. when I start to feel better. I'm not bothered by familiar noises, but unknown noises bother me. I have a 19-year-old son and a 15-year-old daughter. My house is very noisy. I wake up in pain at around 11 p.m.; but I can get up feeling 'well' in the morning, without pain. I take an antispasmodic drug at night.'

This patient says that sometimes, when he is on his balcony at home, he feels as if the world continues to go round, but that he has stopped; he feels desperate, wants to 'go on', but is resigned to the fact that he can't. He feels he has come to the end of the road and feels totally disheartened. In his work as a jeweller, for example, he used to enjoy creating new designs. Now he has no interest in this, and the only thing he does is mount and repair pieces. His creative side is dormant. For this same reason, he has not painted any more pictures for over a year. Creativity had always been a part of his life, but not any more. He used to attend painting lessons but left them a year ago, even though painting was his whole life.

Spiritually, he considers his life is over. He has the intention of continuing with his mission, on other, higher planes. He says that perhaps he will then start to reap what he has sown. According to theosophy, he explains, when an individual physically dies, there is a vital part which assimilates everything that was produced, experienced and achieved during physical life. He maintains that physicality is only a way of moving from one place to the other. He again says that he feels very nervous; he has no time for anyone who approaches him with their troubles, even his son and daughter – something he never did before. He doesn't get angry nor does he insult people, but he regrets the joylessness of his life. He believes he is lucky to have such a good wife (an angel, he says). Whenever his wife sees that he is nervous, she calms and comforts him. His wife is his soulmate; they are very compatible and close. They are together all day long, because he works at home. He says that thanks to his wife he can carry on with his life. If it weren't for her understanding, he would 'go mad'.

He does not want to be bothered with telephone calls and asks his family to say he is not in, even if it is a friend. He will go to the telephone only if his wife asks him to. He has had friends at the Theosophical Society for more than twenty years, who are very fond of him and he of them but he does not want to visit them; but they do sometimes come to see him. Nowadays he does not attend his meetings at the Theosophical Society, in part because he does not want to see his friends. If they ask him to give a talk he will not do it, with the excuse that he is sick. Nevertheless, he feels that a sick person, even with what little health they may have left, must keep on struggling. He does not feel so much defeated as finished, as if he has come to the end of the road. Sometimes at night, when he feels ill, he fears he is dying and takes off his wedding ring and gives it to his wife, so that he can be cremated without his ring. (He also belongs to the Cremation Society.)

He works from home for a jewellery shop, for at least six hours a day. He used to be self-motivated about his work and would go in person to the jewellery shop to do his business negotiations. These days he sends his wife to collect and deliver his work for him. He was never used to feel the cold; but recently has become sensitive to it. He used to wear only a short-sleeved vest in winter but now it is 16°C and he is wearing two sweaters. He has become apathetic and indifferent to everything. When one has been a theosophist one's whole life, he says, one acquires a very special outlook on life. The stabbing pains are unbearable; but he does not want to worry his family by complaining about them.

His workshop is on the flat roof, and he can relax in the sun and fresh air during his lunch break. He likes the fresh country air and the seaside. He says that being by the sea at Mar del Plata makes him forget his pains; but he has not been able to go back there because of his feet. The darkness drives him to despair and the light lifts his spirits.

Because of his theosophical beliefs and ideals, he used to be a vegetarian, but now has developed an aversion to vegetables and his diet consists mainly of boiled beef, no poultry or fish. He has constipation alternating with diarrhoea. In summer he perspires heavily on the face with the intense liver pain which radiates to the heart. When he injects himself with insulin he perspires and his hands tremble.

When his children started school, he decided at the age of thirty-seven to complete his secondary education, so that he would be able to help his children with their work. After graduating from high school at the age of forty he entered the School of Fine Arts. He stayed there for a term then employed someone to give him home tuition.

When asked by Dr Kuperman what his life was like before he became a theosophist, he replies:

> I had always had ideas about life that were different from the rest. When I was 25 years old, I discovered theosophy and natural living. Until then, I had always been very poor. I had gone only to primary school. My mother was a diabetic and had very poor health. I had a miserable childhood; we lived in a tenement house, I went barefoot, I was always in trouble, always angry for some reason. Even though I wanted to continue with my studies, I had to leave school at 14 and start working. I had a very unhappy childhood and adolescence. I had five brothers and sisters. At one time there were eight of us living in a single room; we had very few clothes and sometimes we starved for lack of food. My father was a good man, but very poor.

He says that although he earns very little he believes that money does not buy happiness. He finds happiness in his spiritual beliefs rather than in a material possessions.

Last year, Mr M.B. consulted a theosophist-homoeopath about his depression. He was prescribed Phosphorus and Syzygium as a substitute for insulin (although it really does not actually replace insulin). Later on, this homoeopath prescribed a third remedy. He took all these remedies for a time, but there was no improvement. The homoeopath then advised him to continue taking insulin.

Mr M.B. assures me that he had been healthy until the age of thirty-six. He had been vaccinated as a child and had suffered none of the common childhood diseases. He has had warts on his skin. He used to weigh 130 kilograms although he has never been fat. His weight has now gone down to 87 kilograms.

At home, he prefers to be alone, away from everyone and everything. His family says that he has a habit of harping on other people's mistakes too much and they call him a 'crosspatch'. He says that he has problems with his fifteen-year-old daughter. He has tried to bring her up with a strong sense of morals and does not approve of her coming home late from school because she stayed behind talking to someone. He tells her she is too young to socialise and that she must concentrate on her studies. He tries to control his feelings so that his daughter will not turn against him, but he does wish he could be more assertive. Whenever she talks to a boy he feels 'very disappointed', and insists that this bothers him very much. He never says anything to his wife. He always makes an effort to be very affectionate towards her no matter how angry he is feeling. He understands that it is normal for children to grow up and become independent, but is bothered by the fact that they do not need him any more. His family thinks he interferes too much in their lives and he admits that this might be true.

His wife and sister-in-law share his theosophical views, but his children do not. His daughter feels vexed by his supervision and his moralistic views and gets back at him by making fun of his spiritual ideas. He is concerned about his son, a 'very independent' young man, who pays no attention to his words of warning. He lives his own life and often has angry confrontations with his father. Mr M.B. says that his son does not have the same respect towards him that he had for his own father. When they get on well his son is affectionate towards him; but sometimes he says hurtful things that his father will brood over for days.

He says that his wife on the other hand is an extraordinary woman. 'You don't find women like that any more.'

When he is alone he listens to music; if he listens to or watches an intense drama he feels moved to tears but does not weep. He also feels emotional when he sees a drunkard, a beggar or a poor barefoot child who reminds him of his own childhood.

He is not afraid of being alone; in fact he prefers solitude. When he did not have ulcers on his feet, he used to take long walks alone. He says he has always preferred being alone, and that he is 'not the type who has friends'. He says that the friends he does have seek him out, not the other way round. However, he confesses that he cannot do without his wife's company. When someone comes to visit him he tells his family to say he is not in. He feels good by the seaside but does not like being on the sea. At the invitation of a friend who owned a yacht he climbed aboard once, but as soon as it started to move he had to get off as it made him feel dizzy and nauseous.

When night falls he begins to feel tired and depressed, his worst hours being between 11 p.m. and 3 a.m. And with the short winter days, he feels even worse. He is worried by persistently disagreeable thoughts. His aches and pains are worse for damp. The perforated ulcer on the sole of his foot had been suppurating for twenty years; his brother-in-law, a surgeon, said that it was a miracle that the ulcer had scarred. For years, every time the ulcer became gangrenous, the surgeon would cut out the affected part and apply an ointment. However, ever since he has been seeing Dr Detinis the gangrene has disappeared, the wound has healed, and he now feels some resentment towards his brother-in-law because 'he never really cured him' – all he did was cut away the dead flesh and apply ointment.

Mr M.B. drinks water because he likes the taste of it, but not because he feels thirsty.

He takes offence easily. When he feels offended he is aggravated by consolation and withdraws into himself, ignoring the person who has offended him. Above all, he hates dishonesty; he says that he can tell when people are lying. When someone lies to him he feels that the person 'has died' for him.

The patient's beliefs, feelings, sensations and relationships reveal his deepest dynamic disturbance. In disease, the mental symptoms are the decisive ones. In contrast to case-taking performed for pathological diagnosis, homoeopathic case-taking pays particular attention to the patient's subjective symptoms: that is, those that make up the personality of the patient. These are the key to the chronic disease. To understand a patient's innermost psyche requires that the physician becomes skilled in the art of interviewing, listening attentively, not asking leading questions and eliciting spontaneous accounts. The objective is to understand the patient's personality, by systematically inquiring about his life, activities and sense of purpose. We must always take into account the patient's characteristic totality, adding the general symptoms and modalities of the particular symptoms to the mental symptoms. When there are few well-defined mental symptoms we must base our diagnosis on the general symptoms and modalities, even though the mental state is to a greater or lesser degree fundamental to every clinical picture.

We must strive to understand the patient's innermost depths in order to elicit and thereby know which are the true symptoms. In many cases such as this one, the patient's true symptoms and personality are concealed behind a mask.

Mr M.B. has revealed a lot about himself. After a troubled, poverty-stricken childhood, this intelligent, deep-thinking man embraced the study of theosophy and philosophy – as Aristotle and Thomas Aquinas said, a person's intellectual leanings are dictated by his unique abilities.

His study of theosophy, and later his entry into the Freemasonry, was a quest for spiritual upliftment and meaning, a quest that we all share in one way or another. Mr M.B. believes that the body is the temple of the soul. This is a clear, logical and to a certain degree self-evident concept, because the body is an instrument of life. He believes that when the body dies, life continues its course on other planes of existence.

In spite of these beliefs, he has become indifferent to his friends, avaricious and materialistic, witnessed by the fact that when he thinks he is going to die, he takes his ring off so that it will not go into the grave with him. This is at odds with his theosophical beliefs. He understands intellectually that his children must be independent, but he does not want them to get along without him. He has become selfish, fastidious, irritable and controlling of them. This behaviour is inconsistent with his philosophical principles. It is evident that he is under the influence of a morbid process that is dominating his religious and philosophical beliefs.

This is very important in medicine. A child who changes in temperament, for example, from placid to restless, irritable and bad-tempered, is manifesting symptoms of a tubercular constitution, even though there may not as yet be any signs of pathological disturbance. Mr M.B. came to see me suffering from sensations of heaviness and constriction in the chest, and violent pains in the epigastrium and right-sided hypochondrium. Although he is emphatic that he is not afraid of death, he feels when suffering from the constricting chest pain as if death is approaching. One does not have a premonition of death unless one fears it. He feels he is close to death and has nothing more to look forward to. He does not admit a fear of death because of his theosophical beliefs. Here we have a critical symptom picture which manifests itself at midnight, with the sensation of death and a hidden, denied fear of death.

We must strive to understand what the patient really suffers from, and not be misled by what he or she explicitly tells us. Patients often offer explanations that are nothing more than defence mechanisms because they are not willing to face reality.

Mr M.B.'s symptom picture, then, includes being awakened around midnight with chest pain, great anguish and the feeling that death is approaching. Because of his beliefs he denies his fear of death, but reveals his true feelings in the presentiment of death that accompanies the sensations of constriction and heaviness in the chest.

In clinical practice, consideration must be given to all the elements in a case in order to understand what is unique about the patient, what needs to be cured. This holistic clinical perspective is necessary to highlight the characteristic symptoms. His general physical symptoms are few, but well defined. This is a patient with a marked sensitivity to cold, but who nevertheless needs and feels better for fresh air. For the past eleven years he has had diabetes, inherited from his mother, and even though it has been controlled by insulin he has recurrent ulcers on the foot that tend to become gangrenous. The ulcers are better for hot applications. The clinical examination has not revealed anything important. His diet is apparently normal, his blood pressure 160/100, he has slight pains in the right hypochondrium, some abdominal distension, normal reflexes and a ruddy complexion. But the truly important characteristic of this patient is his approach to life, the tremendous gulf between his lifelong quest for perfection and self-realisation to his current spiritual apathy.

He has turned his back on everything – knowledge, philosophy, art, and above all the striving for altruism and service that is shared by every human soul, that which drives us to sacrifice our personal needs for the sake of the common good. He has become egotistical and indifferent. He can neither study, meditate, write or think; he has become antisocial, irritable, intolerant and fastidious. This formerly free-thinking liberated man now has continual arguments with his children who resent his constant interference in their lives. Once a generous and altruistic man, he has become selfish, avaricious, attention-seeking and demanding, even more so since from the depths of his being he senses the approach of annihilation and death.

Through the destructive dynamic process, this man's symptom picture is characterised by the denial of life and the degeneration of the personality. It is indicative of the destructive process that he asks to be cremated after dying; a request that reveals suicidal and masochistic tendencies. In the innermost depths of his tissues, death and decay are manifest in the ulcers and tendency to gangrene. It can be said that he is dying. When he experiences pain and anguish, which motivated him to come and see me, he experiences both the mental and physical sensations of a pathogenic dynamism.

His symptom picture is the following:

Sensation of death
Indifference
Fastidious
Wicked disposition
Worse after midnight
Worse by cold in general
Desire for open air
Better by open air

After repertorisation we have a group of two, three or four remedies, from which we must decide our diagnosis. In the search for the correct remedy, repertorisation is a means and not an end in itself. Taking into account the grades for each rubric and the pathology of the patient, we are looking for a remedy that has a similar sphere of action. Arsenicum Album and Nux Vomica are high on the list for this case, but with one important difference: Nux Vomica neither makes demands nor desires open air as Arsenicum does.

Kent's *Repertory* lists only Arsenicum Album and Nux Vomica under the rubric 'Fastidious'. However, clinical experience also indicates Carcinosin (2 points), Sepia (1 point), Platinum (1 point), Phosphorus (1 point), Graphites (2 points), Alumina (1 point), Conium (1 point) and Anacardium (2 points). Also, under the rubric 'Wicked disposition', only Cocculus and Curare are mentioned, but Arsenicum (3 points), Belladonna (1 point), Calcarea Carbonica (1 point), Lachesis (3 points), Natrum Muriaticum (3 points) and Nux Vomica (1 point) should also be included.

Arsenicum's sphere of action is very similar to this particular patient's symptom picture. Arsenicum is the most miserly and avaricious remedy of the materia medica, with great anxiety and fear of death. It treats destructive diseases with fetid, acrid and excoriating discharges. (Just as the Phosphorus patient burns and the Natrum Muriaticum patient who dries up, the Arsenicum patient decays.) Arsenicum constantly seeks warmth in order to relieve his sensitivity to cold and dresses warmly, leaving the head exposed to fresh air to relieve the congestion.

Arsenicum's personality is sullen, misanthropic, selfish, avaricious and cowardly. He reacts violently to anyone who challenges his egotism. He is easily offended, rude and irritated by trifles, pernickety and fastidious. He is bitterly critical of other people's behaviour, interfering and obsessed with order and discipline – an outer compensation for the inner state of change. He can never leave well alone and will find fault with a picture hanging on the wall, even if only slightly out of line.

It is clear that Arsenicum's destructive potential mirrors Mr M.B.'s syphilitic disease process at the deepest level of his being.

Therefore, the prescription for this case is one dose of Arsenicum Album 1M.

Chapter 18

The Study of the Materia Medica
(1943)

When studying the materia medica we must absorb the remedies in such a way that we are able to 'see' and 'feel' each one as a whole, so that it is possible to recognise the remedy from different perspectives. Just as we are able to recognise an old friend from the details of their personality, we are able to identify each remedy even when the information is not complete.

To achieve the intuitive skill of the great masters of homoeopathy, we must first make a thorough study of a remedy until it is thoroughly assimilated. To 'feel' a remedy is to know it intuitively. Intuition is a synthesis of the elements acquired by the intellect and therefore one of the higher functions of knowledge. But, no matter how desirable intuition may be, it would be a dangerous error to rely merely on hunches rather than acquiring complete information on the remedy.

The mental characteristics of a remedy must be mastered first. Homoeopathy means individualisation. The individual is a person, and the personality is the mental symptomatology. If the physician had a complete knowledge of the mental symptoms of each remedy, he would have all he needed to make the best prescriptions. For example, before they speak of their symptoms, we may already recognise Pulsatilla in the shy, weepy, emotional, pale, fair-haired, soft-mannered young lady; Sulphur in the ragged philosopher; proud, haughty and irritable Platinum or pale, restless, anxious and death-fearing Arsenicum.

Unfortunately, the mental symptoms of most remedies are not well known. It is impossible to compare remedies such as Thuja, Calcarea Arsenicosa, Natrum Sulphuricum, Kali Sulphuricum and others which have not yet been sufficiently proved, even though they are important and deep-acting remedies.

After mastering the remedy's mental symptoms, the general symptoms and modalities must be studied. Careful attention must be given to the two great modalities of heat and cold, as well as reactions to changes in climate, movement, posture and so on.

After a thorough study of the general symptoms and modalities, food likes and dislikes as well as intolerances are next. Particular symptoms are studied in order to draw attention to the remedy's sphere of action. In this way, for example, we will be able to distinguish between a Belladonna congestion and a Bryonia catarrh.

Finally the keynotes – characteristic, rare and peculiar symptoms – must be memorised. These are important guides to the correct remedy.

It is not my intention here to discuss symptoms of menstruation, general bodily functions, special aggravations, acute states which relate to the remedy under study or psychological or physical causes which may cause a similar symptom picture to appear. There is ample discussion of the hierarchy of symptoms in homoeopathic philosophy, and the books listed below provide excellent information on research into these symptoms.

I recommend the study of one remedy a week, with revision of its characteristics every day and comparisons with other remedies. The remedy should also be compared to other remedies regarding the digestive, circulatory and respiratory systems. In this way, the student will become familiar with each remedy from several different perspectives.

Eventually the homoeopath will replace the orthodox concept of disease with that of well-defined characteristics which individualise the patient.

Each remedy must be studied using different texts. Every author has a personal bias in describing a remedy's remedial action and it is therefore detrimental to rely on any one author. As in daily life, an individual is known in as many ways as the number of friends he has.

The remedy should be studied directly from the provings (or better still from the personal experience) of the great masters as recorded in our materia medica. The following books are highly recommended:

H.C. Allen: *Materia Medica of the Nosodes*
Clarke: *A Dictionary of Practical Materia Medica*
Cowperthwaite: *Materia Medica*
Dunham: *Lectures on Materia Medica*
Hahnemann: *Materia Medica Pura*
Hering: *The Guiding Symptoms of Our Materia Medica* (to be used as a reference book, because it does not give the remedy's personality)
Kent: *Lectures on Homoeopathic Materia Medica*
Lathoud: *Etudes de matière médicale homéopathique*
Nash: *Leaders in Homoeopathic Therapeutics*

Pierce: *Plain Talks on Materia Medica*
Wheeler: *Principles and Practice of Homoeopathy*

Wheeler, Nash and Pierce are easy to read; Kent, Lathoud and Clarke have good descriptions of the mental symptom pictures; Dunham and Cowperthwaite are interesting for comparative materia medica; and Hering, Allen and Hahnemann are reference books which should be read at the end.

A careful study of these books should provide homoeopath with the essence of every remedy so that he or she will be able to recognise them in everyday life.

Chapter 19

Ambra Grisea
(1943)

Ambra Grisea is indicated in premature old age, for a person who at fifty looks eighty, who is dreamy and forgetful, with weakness, trembling, unsteadiness and mental confusion.

This is also a remedy for young people with feeble minds, but not insane. Ambra Grisea jumps from one subject to another, with great mental restlessness, asking one question after another without waiting for an answer, unaware that he has not yet had an answer. There are many cases like these in the modern personality, neurotic with a weak mental state.

Ambra Grisea has depression alternating with excitement or vehemence of temper; indifference to people, joy or sadness; surprise at his indifference. Worse in the morning; wakes in a dreamy state, insane at dusk; vertigo of old people with no modalities; cannot go out on the streets; vertigo on rising in the morning, must wait a while before getting out of bed; worse after eating; must lie down because of the vertigo and weak sensation in the stomach; symptoms after eating; senility; when trying to think or meditate, ideas slip away, cannot concentrate and, sits up and cannot help but dwell upon the most disagreeable things; has hallucinations, visions of horrible faces which keep him awake; business affairs can bring on this state of vertigo, congestion in the head and softening of the brain.

The presence of another person aggravates the symptoms. The patient cannot pass a stool unless the nurse leaves the room. Confusion and embarrassment in the presence of other people with trembling, nervous excitement and vanishing thoughts. Ambra Grisea imagines that his mental faculties are failing and he falls into a state of melancholy and does not want to live; loathes life and wants to die; great sadness and melancholy; sits and cries for days, slowly sinking into a state of insanity or dementia; mental prostration, feeble-mindedness; a bereaved person who is grief-stricken and does not think life is worth living.

Ambra Grisea

Many physical symptoms are aggravated by listening to music; music is intolerable, as if it strikes blows upon the physical body; hammering pains in the spinal column on hearing music; palpitations on hearing music from the slightest exertion or from making the slightest mental exertion, with trembling and starting palpitations that start in the feet, and extend to the whole body, with constriction on breathing.

Chapter 20

Argentum Nitricum
(1955)

To gain a clear clinical perspective of the patient and correctly interpret the proving symptoms it is essential to understand the concept of the totality of symptoms.

Medical orthodoxy views the totality of the organism as a collection of organs and tissues which in turn are made up of an aggregate of cells. According to this view, the unity of the organism is achieved through the regulating function of the nervous system.

However, modern biology supersedes this theory with the Hahnemannian principle of vitalism, affirming that the vital force of the organism governs the functioning of all the organs. In other words, each of the different physicochemical structures which make up an organ has a specific function regarding the totality. Localised reactions express the vital intention of the whole person. All functions are coordinated by an innate vital principle.

Using the physiological analysis of physicochemical structures, organic medicine has concentrated exclusively on the body. But the human being also has drives, instincts and emotions, a temperament, and a vital principle or soul. These do not obey the laws of physico-chemical processes, but the laws of adaptation, cause and effect – a vital purpose which determines the form and behaviour of organisms.

The human being shares this biological substratum with all the higher animals, but also has the ability to make decisions, exercise free will and achieve self-realisation. While the outmoded doctrine of atomism has been superseded by recent advances in nuclear physics, medicine has been unable to deal with the complex phenomenon of the consciousness of the self. The ego has both the power of reasoning and the ability to express emotions, and straddles both the outer world and the soul.

Thus all physical and psychic layers of the human being are intimately related and coordinated aspects of the same vital energy, from physical to spiritual expression.

Soul and spirit together make up the human psyche, which in turn is influenced and nourished by the physical body.

Conflicting impulses and emotions reside in the ego, or id. The ego's erotic and aggressive tendencies are controlled or suppressed by the external world, leading to the development of a conscience or super-ego that starts in the first moments of life and continues to evolve through exposure to censorship, education and cultural dictates.

The ego or id is also the battlefield where the struggle for emotional adaptation to life is played out. The whole human drama of disease and anxiety takes place in the ego, which separates man's primitive nature from spirit and the journey to spiritual transcendence. The result of this struggle is the development of character, which is each person's unique formula for the resolution of conflict. The temperament is a person's way of being – his emotional constitution, and the character is a person's way of doing – his reactions to the environment.

The patient's psyche can be understood by studying the character – the unique formula for dealing with the ego's attempts to balance and control his emotional reactions to the outer world.

In homoeopathy, a symptom is upgraded when it is preceded, in the patient's own words, by the pronoun 'I'. It has been empirically recognised that the ego's reactions to sensations, sensory impressions, emotions, ideas, character and behaviour reveal the pathology of the patient. But the ego has rarely been defined or understood. According to depth psychology, the ego's main functions are to perceive, adapt to and act on reality, and to integrate, harmonise, unify and regulate the soma, psyche and spirit. Thus, if the ego is studied essentially through its relationship with the outer world, then the most important clinical examination is that of the patient's character. Through case-taking and analysis of the ego's reactions and defence mechanisms, the physician gains an invaluable understanding of the patient and the remedy.

We have said that every remedy is capable of producing mental and emotional changes in the personality. The polychrests are deep-acting remedies, because they reach to the centre of the morbid disturbance.

Argentum Nitricum is a syphilitic remedy associated with the deterioration of the nervous system, notably of the cortex, the anatomic location of the ego. But before any lesional damage is noticed the personality of the patient has undergone profound changes. When there is a disruption of the primary function of the ego, the balancing of instinctive needs and external reality, the patient lacks the ability to integrate the different aspects of the personality. In other words, when

143

the ego's regulating function is disturbed, homoeostasis or the synchro-nisation of all vital functions of soma and psyche tends to break down.

This is precisely what happens in Argentum Nitricum patients. The ego is too weak to withstand his aggressive impulses and he feels driven to jump from a height, to jump into the void. He is certain that misfortune will inevitably befall him or that he will suffer from a serious disease, have convulsions, die or go insane. His thoughts, fears, phobias and obsessions are uncontrollable. He believes that when he turns the corner he will faint; his fear that something will happen when he goes somewhere brings on an attack of diarrhoea.

Lachesis projects his feelings of aggression onto the outer world and believes that he is being pursued. Aurum has a strong impulse to commit suicide which brings on much anxiety and feelings of guilt. Argentum Nitricum is helpless and incapable of controlling his im-pulses, and feels overwhelmed by fear, anxiety and restlessness. He is always in a stage of great agitation and hurry, as if he is being pursued by an internal enemy from which he is forever trying to escape.

This is similar to Mercurius, who has impulses to commit murder or suicide at the sight of a knife. Mercurius is in a constant state of rest-lessness and uncertainty; he feels as if guilty of a crime and wants to run away from himself.

He has strong uncontrollable impulses to destroy others and is devoid of any sense of morality. Aurum is a guilt-ridden melancholic, with a strong moral conscience. Lachesis has the paranoid belief that he is pursued by death or under superhuman control. Nitricum Acidum blames other people for his problems. Argentum Nitricum is anxious because of the inability of his ego to withstand the violence of his impulses and fearful of losing all self-control.

But no matter how well we understand the character of the remedy – as it is indeed the best guideline for diagnosis – we must also include the general, functional, somatic characteristics of each remedy.

Mercurius is worse by extreme temperatures, such as the heat of the bed and by perspiration; discharges are fetid and the breath is offensive.

Aurum is sensitive to cold in winter, with a tendency to congestion, oversensitivity of the circulatory system, violent palpitations and hot flushes.

Lachesis is warm-blooded, worse in the spring and from sun, from being shut in, from the suppression of discharges, in the morning after sleep, from constriction and contact.

Nitricum Acidum is cold and feels worse from changes in weather and has irritating, excoriating and fetid discharges and inflammation of the mucous membranes. There are splinter-like sensations. The urine smells like horse urine.

Argentum Nitricum is hot, needs fresh air, and feels worse in a hot, stuffy room. There is aggravation from sweets, with inflammation of the mucous membranes and the digestive system.

The relationship between the mind and the body is an empirical fact; it obeys a logic of its own we can never fully grasp. Character is developed by the conflict between external reality and a person's instinctive, emotions, desires, ambitions and needs. When a person expresses his character, he reacts as a whole human being, in a thoroughly coordinated fashion, without omitting any somatic, emotional or spiritual aspect of his being.

Recent research on the psychodynamic factors which play a role in stomach ulcers indicates that ulcerous patients are characterised by anxiety and an excessive childish dependency. They tend to give up all control and return to a primal state in which they must be fed and cared for like a baby. This is the exact mental syndrome of Argentum Nitricum: fearful, apprehensive and anxious, striving with agitation and hurry to compensate for a basic inability to control his impulses. Argentum Nitricum suffers from ataxia or lack of coordination, first of the psyche, later of the digestive system and finally, syphilitic locomotor ataxia.

Chapter 21

Aurum Metallicum
(1955)

Aurum Metallicum has all the destructive tendencies of a syphilitic remedy.

Psora tends to develop hypofunction, congestion and inflammation. Sycosis's dysfunction takes the form of disorderly cell proliferation. Syphilis, psora and sycosis are the three basic stigmata, miasms or diatheses which afflict the human being. All organic pathology is rooted in these three primary dynamic disturbances.

Pure miasmatic types are rarely seen in clinical practice. Patients will usually manifest symptoms of a prevailing miasm with other underlying morbid tendencies at various stages of development. A patient cannot be said to be syphilitic, only that the current symptom picture is predominantly syphilitic. There are so many possible combinations present in a symptom picture that the constitutional diagnosis must be based on detailed comparisons between symptoms and materia medica; aetiological speculation is out of the question.

The identity of the patient is revealed by the mental symptoms and modalities that reflect his ability to adapt to circumstances.

Although it is useful to be familiar with generic constitutional types – such as Hahnemann's psora, syphilis and sycosis, Grauvogl's hydrogenoid, oxygenoid and carbonitrogenoid types or Nebel's calcarea, sulphur and phosphorus – it is the individual's unique susceptibility to the single remedy that must take precedence.

Classifications of patients as lymphatic, arthritic, tubercular and cancerous – the typologies of Kretschmer and Klages and endocrinologically-oriented schools which relate morphology to temperament – are of statistical value but do not individualise the case. When comparing the patient with the remedy, the physician must bear in mind that although the patient might not have all the characteristics of the remedy, the remedy must have all the characteristics of the patient.

Aurum has a well-defined cardiovascular picture; the aorta and the arteries may be affected, giving rise to hypertension with brain and coronary arteriosclerosis. There is great sadness with valvular heart disease.

He is usually stout, sanguine and apopleptic. As seen in Lachesis, Sulphur and Carbo Vegetabilis cases, Aurum has a hot, red, congested and bloated face with rushes of blood to the head. The nose is red and thick with abnormal dilation of arteries and capillaries as seen in cardiac patients and alcoholics with acne rosacea.

In addition to plethora, congestion, heaviness and sluggishness, there is a tendency to jaundice.

Although Aurum's most important symptom is suicidal depression, this symptom is rarely revealed in the interview. In any case, suicidal thoughts is not a characteristic symptom of this remedy.

We must ask ourselves why the patient wants to commit suicide. What has influenced him to make that decision? Usually the person who talks about commiting suicide will not actually do it and the person who does not talk about it is likely to do it. So we must be open to the idea of suicide during the interview and try to understand the psychological factors involved.

As we have mentioned before, homoeopathy connects the body and the mind. Both modern psychiatry and psychosomatic medicine acknowledge that the mental symptoms reveal the human being's innermost depths, his subconscious drives and the inner meaning of his pathology. The homoeopathic remedy acts dynamically on the mental and emotional disturbances which always accompany pathology and encompasses the whole individual.

According to Kent, the will, the instinct of self-preservation, is the core of the human being. He talks about the biological will or vital impulse which emerges from the organism's innermost depths, as distinct from conscious rational mind, that grapples with the problem of free will. Biological will holds the dynamic potential for feelings and emotions, instinctive reactions or subjective experiences which, even though they pertain to consciousness, have little to do with reason or the intellect. This is what the physician must grasp in order to understand the essential dynamic substratum of the patient's disease.

Unlike other psychological processes, the emotions fluctuate between the two extremes of pleasure and displeasure, depression and excitement, tension and relaxation. It is impossible to arrive at a purely objective or rational explanation of the emotions. Subjective knowledge is existential and therefore beyond the reach of objective science. But the fact is that physical symptoms reflect the emotions and can be accurately measured, for example, by lie detectors.

The instincts of eroticism and aggression are essential components of emotion. When these instincts are suppressed by society or by moral conscience, the feelings associated with these instincts are disturbed. According to each person's susceptibility, emotions such as fear, resentment, hate, jealousy, envy, stubbornness, desperation, suspicion and sadness may arise, as well as other more socially unacceptable feelings and reactions such as pride, vanity, dishonesty and avarice. These mental symptoms are clinically useful.

The individuality of the patient refers to the extent to which his feelings or emotions have been inhibited by parents, and social and cultural norms, which is why he is always effected emotionally by the people in his life. Feelings and emotions play a large part in the relationships between human beings. Just as it makes little sense to study liver function in isolation from the whole body, the patient must be considered in relation to his environment.

And just as the modalities of sensation, aggravation, amelioration and time qualify a symptom, feelings and emotions further enable the physician to individualise the case.

The patient's feelings, experiences and emotions reveal the point of causation of pathology. Thus, from a clinical point of view, a detailed case history is most important. The proving and clinical symptoms of Aurum allow the physician to understand the emotional causation of the suicidal disposition.

Aurum is basically an irritable, irascible patient who is intolerant of contradiction and has violent outbursts of uncontrollable, destructive rage. Rage and anger are turned inwards, manifesting as depression and self-hatred. Melancholy is the state which precedes the idea of suicide, an idea which the patient will rarely admit to harbouring. The psychological components of this depression are guilt, self-condemnation and self-reproach. Aurum is the most destructive and anxious of the syphilitic remedies, full of self-hatred and despair, helpless, and unworthy of consideration and kindness. He believes that he has lost the affection of friends and family, and constantly laments and prays for forgiveness. He is taciturn, melancholy and hypochondriacal, and his self-hatred may cause him to jump from the balcony.

He feels like a criminal and will lash out in anger at the slightest offence or contradiction. The symptom picture is one of aggression, manic depression and self-destruction.

'One of these days I will kill all of you and kill myself', he exclaims in his violent moments. The newspapers are full of stories like these.

Incapable of containing the violence of his emotions, Aurum reacts intensely to a fright, a disappointed love, the loss of a loved one, contradiction, anger in an argument, mortification or vexation. The symptom picture is one of fear, anxiety, trembling, palpitations, angina, thoracic contriction, despair, weeping, melancholy and, finally, suicide. In the words of Hahnemann, great anxiety culminating in ideas of suicide with spasmodic constriction of the lower abdomen.

Aurum is also restless, agitated, wants to do things quickly as if time were running out, with a sensation of vertigo, a feeling of congestion and heat in the head, with cold hands and feet, as if all the blood would flow to the head or as if a rush of hot air would run through the head. Two essential modalities of this remedy are the desire for open air to cool the face and all symptoms are worse at night – a characteristic of the syphilitic miasm.

Aurum is the most destructive of all syphilitic remedies and the most profoundly depressed. Aurum's aggression, anger and indignation are of secondary importance to the feelings of guilt and remorse, the despair of salvation (religious), self-reproach and suicidal thoughts. There is also the fear of insanity, hysteria and obsessive behaviour which characterise other remedies from the materia medica.

Aurum, Arsenicum, Psorinum, Medorrhinum, Mercurius, Alumina, Chelidonium and Digitalis all have suicidal impulses, the fear of death, and a terrible anxiety of conscience as if guilty of a crime.

Arsenicum is a weak, prostrated patient whose vitality has been wasted away by chronic ill health, the strains and stresses of life, and internal toxicity. It has intense irritability, profound anxiety, agitation and despair. The fear of death rises from the depths of Arsenicum's exhausted organism.

Psorinum also fears death, is very sad, depressed and pessimistic, despairs of getting well, and lacks the vitality to react to acute disease. Psorinum's attacks of anger, anxiety and melancholy make life intolerable for himself and his loved ones. He feels the cold, is dirty and foul-smelling, with itchy skin eruptions.

Medorrhinum feels as if guilty of an unforgivable sin. Like Aurum, Medorrhinum is agitated, impatient and fearful, but the salient features of this remedy are the fear of the dark and of insanity, the poor memory and sycotic ailments such as pelvic infections, rheumatism, chronic catarrh and enlarged glands.

Alumina has great mental confusion with defective reasoning faculties are impaired. He feels so disorientated that he doubt his identity, believing that he has transferred to another person everything which he perceives or feels. Sensations are transmitted very slowly to

149

the nerve centres. The thoughts are disordered; there is progressive paralysis. He feels guilty as if of a crime and has a violent impulse to commit suicide upon seeing blood or a knife.

Chelidonium is sad, depressed and melancholy, also with an anxiety of conscience as if having committed a crime or unpardonable sin, and feels he has been eternally condemned.

Basically Chelidonium is irritable, passionate and quarrelsome, and has violent fits of rage. As in Lycopodium, Chelidonium's mental state is associated with liver dysfunction with two basic keynotes: pain in the right shoulder blade and drowsiness on awakening and after meals.

The action of Digitalis on the liver is similar to Chelidonium. Digitalis has manic outbursts of rage followed by a deep melancholy, weeping and fear of death. The prevailing symptom in this remedy is anxiety of conscience.

Mercurius is not as violent as Aurum. However, Mercurius has great restlessness and agitation with impulses to kill or to commit suicide. He has an unconscious fear of himself and wants to run far away.

Mercurius is characterised by great restlessness and uneasiness, which prevents him from staying still in any one place, especially at night. Mercurius is like a delinquent criminal.

Other remedies with a tendency to suicide are: Natrum Sulphuricum, Calcarea Carbonica, Capsicum, China, Cimicifuga, Hepar Sulphuris, Hyoscyamus, Kali Bromatum, Lac Defloratum, Lachesis, Nux Vomica, Plumbum, Pulsatilla, Sepia, Spigelia, Stramonium and Zincum. However, these remedies do not have the feelings of guilt and self-hatred that are characteristic of the preceding remedies.

While Mercurius, Alumina, Arsenicum and Natrum Sulphuricum all have a fear of acting out their suicidal impulses, Aurum does not. In Mercurius the emphasis is on the desire to commit murder; in Aurum, it is the desire to commit suicide.

The suicidal thoughts of Natrum Sulphuricum are not due to anxiety of conscience as in Aurum. Natrum Sulphuricum is weak, apathetic, deeply depressed and so weary of life that he does not want to live. This remedy has the sycotic aggravation in the morning, sensitivity to wet weather, migraine, oedemas, catarrh and asthma.

The loss of self-confidence of Aurum, Anacardium, Calcarea Fluorica, Kali Phosphoricum, Lycopodium, Pulsatilla, Psorinum and Silica finds its expression through a range of symptoms, from shyness to pride.

Anacardium is depressed, forgetful, irresolute and ambivalent about his constant conflict between desire and duty.

Calcarea Fluorica is also indecisive and overwhelmed by fears and financial worries, like Psorinum, who also fears financial ruin or failure in business ventures.

Kali Phosphoricum is tired, weak-willed and highly-strung, too exhausted to work.

Pulsatilla has a feminine temperament, is sweet, passive, lacks self-confidence, and does not have the slightest aggression.

Silica has no backbone, is chilly, oversensitive and easily discouraged.

On a physical level, Aurum is a remedy for chronic syphilitic cases that have been suppressed by the use of mercury. It is indicated in cardio-vascular disease with circulatory problems and arteriosclerosis (as opposed to Plumbum's nephritic disease); indurations of the glands, as in orchitis, fibromas, caries of the bones, ozaena and diseases of the eye such as retinitis and detached retina.

Head

Vertigo as if spinning round in a circle when bending down or when rising from the lying position. Feels as if drunk when walking in open air. Tendency to lean or fall to the left side.

Mental work produces brain-fag with throbbing pains.

Sensation of a rush of air through the head if it is not warmly wrapped. Hot, plethoric, congested head. Bloated face; sees stars.

Severe pains in the bones; periostitis and exostosis of the cranial bones, worse at night.

Hair falls out, especially in syphilis.

Eyes

Increase of pressure in the eyeballs. Glaucoma with pains upon pressure and diminished vision. Veil before the eyes. Heat, burning sensation and red eyes. Retinitis, protruding eyeballs.

Vertical hemiopia. Sees darkness or the upper half of the visual field. Lycopodium and Lithium Carbonicum also have hemiopia, but they see the right half of objects.

Ears

Chronic fetid suppuration of the ears with caries of the mastoid process. Very sensitive to noise, but better by music.

Swollen tonsils bring on dullness of hearing. Humming and cracking in the ears.

Nose

Thick, swollen, red nose with scaly eruptions. Nasal malignancy. Congestion with acute sense of smell followed by loss of sense of smell. Ozaena. Rhinitis with yellowish-green secretion, crusty and fetid or like egg-white and morning catarrh.

Teeth

Toothache, worse at night and when breathing in cold air.

Mouth

Halitosis; foul breath at puberty.
Necrosis of the bones of the hard palate. Ulcers on the gums. Excessive salivation. Pains worse at night.

Appetite

Increased; bulimia and thirst. Aversion to meat (as in syphilis).

Stomach

Acid, burning sensation, regurgitation. Pains upon lightly touching the epigastrium.

Abdomen

Aurum is an important liver remedy. Anger with yellow bile and melancholy with black bile.
Aritaeus of Cappadocia, who lived in the first and second centuries A.D., first postulated the theory that both mania and melancholy were both located in the right hypochondrium. A forerunner of today's concept of manic-depressive disorders.
Enlarged, swollen, inflamed liver with burning pains.
Tense, distended abdomen, with rumbling in the bowels, flatulent colic and colicky stools.
Tendency to hernias and bile.
Nocturnal diarrhoea with burning sensation or constipation with small stools.

Urinary System

Polyuria in hypertensive patients. Turbid, milky urine with copious, mucous sediment. Albuminuria.

Male Sexual Organs

Sexual desire greatly increased with or without erections. Nocturnal emissions, priapism. Prostatic fluid without erections. Indurated testes, generally the right testicle, painful to the touch. Hydrocele. Atrophy of the testes in children.

Female Sexual Organs

Abdominal pains as if menses were about to appear. Indurated and prolapsed uterus. Ailments of the uterus; with depression and suicidal thoughts. Amenorrhoea or scanty, late menses. Profuse, corrosive, acrid, thick leucorrhoea, worse from walking. Jaundice during pregnancy and deep melancholic depression.

Respiratory System

Asthma attacks at night or in open air. Cardiac asthma. Sensation of constriction in the chest. Morning cough with viscous yellowish catarrh upon awakening.

Heart and Circulatory System

Congestion of the chest, with palpitations, anxiety, great oppression and hot flushes. Angina extending to the left arm. Enlarged heart with a sensation of fullness. Heart feels as if it would stop, has irregular heart-beat and violent palpitations.

While walking, sensation of heart beating in chest as if it were loose.

As in Kali Carbonicum, Aurum is aggravated by motion.

Raised blood pressure. (Clinical experience shows that manic-depression is usually accompanied by high blood pressure.)

Back and Extremities

Inflammation of the bones with back pain. Periostitis, exostosis and chronic effects of mercury treatment in syphilitic patients. At night and on waking has sensation of paralysis in the limbs. Paralysis, pain and weakness in the knees; feels as if there were a tight bandage around the knees. Sharp, cramping pains in the smaller joints of the hands and feet.

General Symptoms and Modalities

Great plethora of blood with congestion of the head and chest, palpitations of the heart and hot flushes. Aurum can also have chilliness with cold hands and feet. Sensitive to cold, but seeks open air to relieve congestion. All symptoms worse at night, from sunset to sunrise. Right side predominates.

Chapter 22

Kali Carbonicum
(1955)

The characteristic of this remedy is a fear of solitude with an aversion to consolation.

The remedy cries constantly, from intense anxiety that she will die; cries without cause and while sleeping.

There is much anxiety and apprehension in the stomach; she has sad premonitions about the future, fears of disease and of being incurable; easily frightened, starts when touched and on hearing noise; aversion to being touched; screams with fright at an imagined apparition; irritable and bad-tempered after a vexation; offended by trifles; intolerant of the slightest noise; impatient with her children; easily roused to anger and violence especially if things do not turn out as she wants them to; hurried and hyperactive.

Kali Carbonicum is capricious and subject to conflicting desires and fluctuating moods, at times calm, quiet and optimistic, at other times annoyed by trifles and despairing.

This remedy is useful in such conditions as asthma, bronchitis, pulmonary affections, anaemia with tubercular manifestations, female genital affections with Sepia-like characteristics and nervous hysteria.

Kali Carbonicum patients are lymphatic, phlegmatic types, with relaxed tissues, lax fibre and a tendency to obesity. They have a dysfunctional water with pallor, anaemia and great debility due to poor muscle tone.

They are very sensitive to cold, have a profuse perspiration and tend to develop oedemas, especially of the inner upper eyelid.

Kali Carbonicum patients have sudden flushings of the face, hot flushes and palpitations. They are always fatigued, with weakness of the muscles and myocardium. They have thick skin with oedematous swelling.There is a sensation of heaviness in the sacrolumbar region. Farrington characterises Kali Carbonicum with the following triad: perspiration – lumbago – weakness.

They are bad-tempered, impatient, discontented – antagonistic and moody. Their discontent arises from a profound sense of physical and mental weakness, which renders them incapable of coping with life and puts them in a very dependent situation. They are timid, full of fears and apprehensions about the future, death, disease and life itself.

Like everyone else, Kali Carbonicum would like to be free from all dependency but, because she attempts to affirm this aggressively, much anxiety is aroused.

Irritated by her weakness, Kali Carbonicum becomes angry at everything, is sensitive to the slightest unexpected noise, to the slightest touch, especially on the feet. Kali Carbonicum's sensitivity to noise extends even to the human voice; she does not want to hear anyone talking, and desperately runs home to draw peace and comfort from her partner.

This is a tubercular constitution. Debility, anaemia and muscular weakness are common in asthmatic and other respiratory conditions. The asthmatic patient is generally a debilitated individual whose personality is not strong enough to deal with the outer world.

At the root of every asthmatic, says Alexander, there is always an underlying fear of separation from the mother or surrogate mother-figure – someone to depend upon emotionally, who carries out a mother's loving and protecting role. The fear of offending this maternal figure is precisely what occurs in Kali Carbonicum, an excellent remedy for asthma.

This is a fearful, hypersensitive and aggressive remedy that starts at the slightest sound, anxiety tends to take the form of asthma attacks (weeping of the lungs); anguish is felt in the pit of the stomach, the seat of this remedy's functional susceptibility.

Weakness and irritability reflect the remedy's fluctuations between fear and anger, apprehension and aggression, dependency and rebellion.

The remedy has stabbing, piercing burning pains that wander around the body. The nerves are extremely sensitive to cold, even to the slightest draught. Pains are felt in the exposed parts of the body.

As with other hydrogenoid remedies such as Natrum Sulphuricum and Thuja, Kali Carbonicum's symptoms are worse from 2 to 5 a.m. – a time of increased humidity.

Worse after coition, with lumbar pains, general debility, weak vision and trembling.

Worse lying on the left side or on the painful side, in contrast to Bryonia, who feels better for pressure on the affected side.

Kali Carbonicum is passive, timid and cowardly, irritable and sensitive to sensory stimuli. This contradictory pattern is commonly seen in asthmatics, and arises from the need for and the fear of losing maternal affection and support.

However, this analysis of the asthmatic personality is purely theoretical and asthma is not just a psychosomatic condition. It is a combination of constitutional, neurological, psychological and environmental allergenic factors. This holds true in all cases of allergies.

As we all know, asthma is not necessarily cured by identifying or suppressing the allergen. Since Richet's discovery of anaphylaxis, recognition has grown of the importance of emotional factors in hypersensitivity.

Recent neurological research has revealed that olfactory stimuli such as dust, wool, flowers and pollen affect the rhinencephalon, and consequently the emotions. A chronic emotional situation is capable of sensitising the encephalic centres rendering them susceptible to olfactory allergens.

With the strong need to be loved and emotionally supported by a maternal figure, asthmatics often become very attached to those physicians who inspire confidence in their patients and show 'maternal' concern for their welfare. Thus the psyche and the nervous system play a very important role in asthma attacks.

The conventional approach to the treatment of asthma acknowledges the need for desensitising medication and an awareness of the psychological issues, but it fails to address the other important factors which influence the asthmatic patient's constitution.

Hahnemann states that the physician must be objective and non-judgmental in order to understand the patient in the light of his whole life history, both emotional and pathological. The physician must strive to understand the dynamics between the patient and his disease.

Every patient has emotional disorders, problems of conscience, emotional maladjustment and conflicts with people. The physician must know about these situations, not only in order to make a diagnosis, but because, in telling his story and gaining unexpected awareness of his unconscious motivations, the patient comes to understand himself better. Even though they may not be expert psychoanalysts, every physician must know how to listen and ask questions in a non-invasive manner. The homoeopath can then understand and distinguish constitutional symptoms from the mental symptoms that are related to the patient's environment.

The mothers of asthmatic children are often strong, dominating figures who force the child into a subordinate role. During the consultation, these shy and frightened children will continually look to their mothers for approval. Their food preferences, and other likes and dislikes, are likely to be strictly controlled by their mothers.

Psychoanalytic theory contends that these children fear rejection or abandonment by the mother if they were to express strong feelings towards her.

It is common knowledge that the asthmatic symptom picture develops at the age of four or five, after several bouts of colds and bronchitis.

Adult men tend to see their wives as surrogate mothers, thus perpetuating the position of emotional dependence throughout their lives.

With the physician's support, the patient can acknowledge such repressed hostility and fear of the person on whom they are emotionally dependent and can begin to understand their own inner conflict.

This syndrome is common to asthmatics, and is also seen in ulcer patients (such as Argentum Nitricum), but must be individualised using the modalities of the remedy.

It can be said that all asthmatics are timid and need compassion and consolation. Allergy patients have a strong need to be loved, especially by the mother or mother-figure.

However, the physician must be able to distinguish between Lachesis's projection of inner feelings onto the outer world, Lycopodium's defence mechanism, Natrum Sulphuricum's disgust with life, Psorinum's ingrained pessimism, Sulphur's hyperactive egotism, Thuja's obsessive behaviour, Silica's obstinacy and inadequacy, and Kali Carbonicum's sensitivity to stimuli and offences.

An asthmatic patient could require any constitutional remedy. The point is, the physician must look beyond the asthmatic syndrome and psychogenic influences in the patient's environment. The constitutional remedy will perform better if the obstacles to cure in the patient's environment are also removed or lessened.

Mental Symptoms

Desire for company. Depression and sadness. Despair.
Anxious foreboding at dusk.
Full of fears. Apprehension and fear of being alone.
Fear of being incurable. Fear of disease.
Apprehension in stomach.
Disagreeable mood. Stubborn, does not know what he or she wants.
Demanding, not satisfied with anything.
Fear of work.
Difficulty concentrating.

Irresolute.

Wakes with a start in the middle of the night, speaks to spouse and later does not remember anything.

Feels as if thoughts were vanishing. Absent-minded.

Cannot find the correct words to express thoughts. Makes mistakes when speaking.

Frequent state of confusion with loss of consciousness.

Sensation of mental confusion, dullness, stupefaction, as if intoxicated.

Stomach: after excitement. Things are felt in the stomach.

Apprehension in stomach: Asaf., Aur., Bry., Calc., Cann. Sat., Canth., Dig., Kali C., Lyc., Mez., Phos., Thuja.

Weeps when telling her symptoms: Kali C., Med., Puls., Sep., Sil.

Chapter 23

Lachesis
(1955)

The homoeopath must strive to understand the physical and mental characteristics of each remedy. The mental and emotional symptoms are the best guide, revealing as they do the nerve centre of the remedy.

It is on this plane of central, hypothalamic and sensory activity that we find each remedy's personal character. The pathogenesis yields the mental syndrome which we must strive to grasp.

Lachesis's most salient general symptoms are:

1) Aggravation after sleep.
2) Oversensitive to touch and constriction.
3) Left side predominates or symptoms travel from left to right.
4) Amelioration from discharges.
5) Intolerance of heat and enclosed spaces.

Lachesis suffers from melancholy, fear, premonitions of death, irritability, excitement, loquacity and jealousy. How then can we gain a true understanding of this remedy's mental symptoms?

The following schema is useful for understanding the patient's personality and the remedy's underlying emotional dynamics.

The human being has a desire for both pleasure and destruction, eroticism and aggression, each of which create tension and are vital for self-preservation.

These impulses are the source of all our drives, feelings and emotions. The external world inhibits their expression through moral norms and censorship, and the result is a constant conflict between the primitive self and the external world.

Health can be defined as a state of perfect harmony between what a person requires from life and what the world can realistically offer him. Disease, then, is the expression of unmet needs. In cases of allergy, for example, this vital imbalance underlies the psoric oversensitivity, the syphilitic aggression, and destruction and the sycotic overstimulation and hyperfunction.

159

The presence of a harmful agent, emotion, trauma, germ or toxin triggers the susceptibility to disease according to the individual's unique group of unfulfilled needs. Once the mind and body have been activated in this way, they react according to the organism's unique functional disturbance with modalities that are individual to the patient.

Lachesis Trigonocephalus, the poison from the terrible surukuku snake, is a remedy that produces a symptom picture similar to that of patients affected by depression, vexation, grief, long-term emotional breakdown, septic infection, and intoxication.

The remedy's mental symptoms are well defined. Hering states that this poison finds its best prover in a melancholic subject.

As in all provings, the primary reaction is an exacerbation of the latent conflict between the primitive self and the dictates of society. This gives rise to the person's unique formula for conflict resolution. Predominantly syphilitic remedies tend to heighten aggression; predominantly sycotic remedies tend to intensify sexual perversions.

Lachesis is malicious, proud, cutting, suspicious and fault-finding. This symptom picture is typical of menopausal women going through a personality crisis brought on by hormonal changes.

They have a fear of the unknown and of death, especially of death coming during sleep. As a defence mechanism, a Lachesis woman projects her fears and believes she is under the influence of a malignant, superior power, that she is pursued by enemies who try to grab her or kill her, that she has been harmed or hexed, that there are burglars in the house, that the very remedy she takes is poison or even that her own family is preparing her funeral because she will surely die.

Her own hostility towards others is projected in such a paranoid, persecuting manner that she falls into a melancholy state with much sighing. A Lachesis woman fearfully isolates herself from other people, has no desire to talk, doubts everything, does not trust anyone and refuses to get involved in the world. Apathetic and weary of life, she feels extremely sad and lonely on waking in the morning, feeling devoid of affection or friends, and longs for death.

A strong characteristic of this remedy is the projection of the patient's fear and anger onto others. The Lachesis patient is convinced that she is a target for all the world's evil, and is oversensitive and extremely suspicious of what people say, albeit with the best of intentions. Whether the patient is a menopausal women or a man at a critical age, Lachesis will transfer their own desires for conjugal infidelity onto their spouse, thus giving rise to violent and dramatic jealousy, with angry reproaches and insults, sneers, cutting sarcasm and an endless stream of absurd and ridiculous insinuations.

Their loquacity causes them to jump quickly from one idea to the next; from one subject to another, led by a word which brings to mind the most disparate topics, which they then follow without completing the phrase.

The Lachesis mental syndrome, then, has as a defence mechanism extreme mental activity with uncontrollable loquacity and the projection of fear, anger and sexuality onto others.

During attacks or aggravations, which usually occur at nightfall, Lachesis may become delirious, chattering constantly. The face is red and bloated; there is much difficulty in pronouncing words correctly. Anything tight or even the touch of clothing may be unbearable. After a quarrel due to jealousy, for example, Lachesis is the image of the furious woman who, face on fire, eyes popping out of their sockets and insults bubbling out of her mouth, places her hand on her chest and sinks into unconsciousness.

The hyperactivity, hypersensitivity and tendency for projection is a typical spiritualist symptom picture. Extrasensory phenomena are interpreted as images, hallucinations and experiences that involve hearing, smelling and touching, or muscular actions such as automatic writing and the use of the pendulum or divining rod.

Lachesis can have clairvoyant abilities such as dowsing or being able to detect metals. Lachesis women may even think that they are someone else in the hands of a superior power, that they are under the control of a superhuman force or that they are dead and their body is being used by spirits.

Chapter 24

Lycopodium
(1955)

Lycopodium is thought to be the first plant on earth. The remedy comes from a plant that has been on the earth for six hundred million years. Previously a tree, it is today a type of moss.

The remedy has liver problems that can lead to chronic toxaemia. Symptoms may present as the mildest indigestion or irreversible liver and kidney damage – all degrees of intensity and variations are possible in its symptom picture.

General Appearance

A cursory examination will reveal a pale and yellowish or copper-like complexion, darker at the temples. Deep lines and furrows, especially between the eyebrows and on the forehead, give the patient a prematurely aged look. The eyes are lively and intelligent, but sunken and surrounded by a bluish areola due to venous stasis.

Lycopodium is easily embarrassed, shy and tongue-tied, but once he gains confidence he becomes self-possessed and speaks with a rather bitter vehemency. He feels discouraged by his increasing physical and mental inadequacy. During the consultation, restless Lycopodium constantly shifts in the chair, his face contorted by spasmodic tics and grimaces.

This is a grim, bitter, irritable and suspicious neurotic who shuns other people's sympathy. Sceptical and bored, Lycopodium patients will invariably describe a long history of various ineffective treatments for digestive and intestinal disorders and emotional problems.

Physical Examination

A striking feature of the remedy is the shape of Lycopodium's body. The face, neck and upper trunk are thin and emaciated, while the lower body is disproportionately broad. The abdomen is protruding and flaccid and the legs have oedematous varicose veins. This peculiar body shape is reminiscent of Natrum Muriaticum, as compared with Abrotanum and Argentum Nitricum, who have thin legs with a large thorax and thick-set face.

The skin is as dry as parchment, poorly nourished, and yellowish. Often there are eczematous eruptions, sometimes itchy, as well as naevi, freckles, copper-like blotches and spider spots on the face as seen in alcoholic cases. Bromidrosis of the feet and armpits is usually present.

The enlarged liver, seen more frequently in China cases, is easy to detect by touching the patient's round and distended abdomen. Both hypochondria are painful to the touch and there is often a gurgling sound in the right iliac fossa. There is a tendency to low blood pressure.

Following the usual order in which patients reveal their symptoms – after the physician has won the patient's confidence – we shall leave this remedy's subjective, mental symptoms until the end. Mental symptoms such as pride, rudeness, jealousy and avarice are obviously not disclosed immediately by the patients themselves and therefore require a reasonable period of time in order to be gleaned through subtle and attentive observation.

Lycopodium acts on the digestive, respiratory and urinary systems, provoking a catarrhal condition which alternates with dryness of the mucous membranes.

Digestive System

All Lycopodium patients have a dyspeptic symptom picture, but in some cases it may be masked by general symptoms, especially when irritability, mental inability or loss of memory are so marked that they alarm the patient. The lips are dry with herpetic eruptions, as seen in Natrum Muriaticum, Sepia and Rhus Tox. The mouth is dry and thirstless like Pulsatilla. Spasms of the throat and oesophagus also occur, as well as pain behind the mid sternum caused by trapped gas. Lycopodium has sluggish digestion and, according to Kent, a ravenous appetite like Iodum.

The following are black type rubrics in Kent. The appetite increases with eating. As in Phosphorus, Psorinum and China, these patients will get up at night to eat. They crave sweets like Argentum Nitricum, China and Sulphur, and onions like Thuja, and oysters like Lachesis, although both onions and oysters aggravate.

The most important digestive symptom is easy satiety. Soon after starting to eat, Lycopodium patients feel so full that they stop eating, loosen their clothing, especially around the epigastrium, and try to eructate. While Natrum Muriaticum has indigestion, Lycopodium suffers from an acid stomach, heartburn and regurgitations.

The abdomen is tympanitic with audible gurgling and pain, especially in the splenic angle of the colon; there is also diffuse pain in the right hypochondrium. Lycopodium tends to have trapped gas in the intestines, while Carbo Vegetabilis has trapped gas in the stomach and China in both the intestines and the stomach.

This remedy has constipation and ineffectual urging. The Silica and Alumina constituents of Lycopodium are responsible for the dry mucous membranes and sluggish bowels. The ineffectual urging of Nux Vomica is caused by antiperistaltic contractions, whereas in Lycopodium it is caused by ineffective expulsion reflexes of the sphincter.

Respiratory System

The homoeopath must distinguish between the symptoms of the disease, which are common to all patients, and the particular symptoms of the patient. For example, a patient may present with chills (which we know to be the result of a rise in temperature in the centre of the organism), congestion and the draining of blood from the surface, which causes pallor and shivering. When body temperature rises to the surface, there is congestion of the skin and the organism attempts to cool itself through profuse perspiration, and the resultant dehydration produces thirst.

Although symptoms such as these are useful for identifying a syndrome, they do not help us individualise a particular patient. However, if we find that a patient has fever with copious sweating and dehydration of the mucous membranes, a dry mouth but no thirst, this can be considered to be a rare, peculiar symptom, unique to this particular patient.

A particular characteristic of Lycopodium is the fan-like movement of the outer ends of the nostrils from muscular contractions, which may also cause facial tics and cramps in the calves. There is toxaemia of the muscles, especially of the smaller muscles, the contractile fibres of the hollow organs such as the intestines and blood vessels and orifices such as the nasal fossae and the anus.

In Lycopodium the twitching of the nostrils is not associated with respiratory difficulties as seen in acute lung disease. Antimonium Tartaricum, Phosphorus and Sulphur are some of the remedies that share this symptom, but it is most marked in Lycopodium. When seen in a nursing infant with an acute lung disorder, this symptom is especially important. The eyes remain half-open during sleep, due to problems with the contraction reflexes.

Lycopodium suffers from a very stuffy nose at night. The nasal discharge is a purulent mucus that forms elastic plugs when dry, as in Kali Bichromicum. Lycopodium children wake up at night with snuffles like Ammonium Carbonicum, Nux Vomica or Sambucus, and scratching their noses like Arum Triphyllum.

There is copious tracheobronchial catarrh, with purulent mucus. Lycopodium may be indicated in patients with right-sided lobar pneumonia who are slow to recover. They have a cough and digestive problems, and have never been well since a bout of pneumonia.

Genital and Urinary System

The acidic urine produces a burning sensation in the urethra. There are stones in the kidneys and gallbladder due to excessive amounts of oxalates, urates and uric acid.

The urine has red sand-like sediment. As in Sarsaparilla and Borax, Lycopodium children cry before urinating. Like Lachesis, headaches and gouty pains increase when the thick, yellowish nasal discharge is suppressed and the urine is clear, indicating that toxins are not being cleared from the organism.

Other symptoms are urine retention, polyuria and enuresis; impotence with depression; painful coitus in women due to dryness of the mucous membranes and pains and lesions of the right ovary.

Modalities

Lycopodium has three well-defined modalities: right side predominates; worse between 4-6 p.m. or 4-8 p.m.; and sensitive to but better by cold.

All inflammation and pain begins on the right side and travels from right to left. So Lachesis, a complementary and left-sided remedy, can cure a case started by Lycopodium.

Lycopodium feels worse 4-8 p.m., with the peak aggravation at 6 p.m. After 8 p.m. he either makes a drastic recovery or remains ill throughout the evening.

In a healthy state, the organism tends to be active from the morning until early afternoon; later on, vital activity begins to wind down as evening approaches. This rhythm is seen in Lycopodium, with the early evening aggravation coming at a time when it is normal to feel tired.

It is important to differentiate between the symptom of aggravation at certain specific times and the worsening of symptoms due to normal tiredness at the end of an active day. Of course, any reversal or alteration of the normal vital rhythm should be especially noted. The evening aggravation of Lycopodium is caused by liver dysfunction during digestion.

Lycopodium patients are cold, slow and weak. The digestive problems produce venous stasis and congestion in the brain, causing aggravation from enclosed spaces and stuffy rooms, and amelioration from fresh air that relieves the sensation of blood pulsating in the head. As in Apis, Bryonia, Iodum, Pulsatilla, Kali Sulphuricum and Sulphur, Lycopodium is worse from the heat of the bed and from being in a closed space.

While Silica is better from keeping the head warm, these patients cannot bear to have their heads covered.

The head and spinal column are better for fresh air, all other symptoms are relieved by heat in general. The throat and stomach are better for hot drinks and hot food, pains and inflammations are relieved by hot packs. Like Arsenicum, Lycopodium patients wrap up excessively but also like to feel cool air on their face and head to relieve congestive headaches.

Although Phosphorus is much more sensitive to cold than Lycopodium the overactive metabolism of the former causes the patient to 'burn' from internal combustion, so to speak, thus producing the craving for cold food and drink.

Lycopodium has a sluggishness of the venous system, the portal vein, capillaries and coeliac artery all being affected. Like Pulsatilla, Ferrum, Kali Sulphuricum, Rhus Tox., Sepia and Sulphur, Lycopodium is better from motion, which stimulates the circulation, provided the patient does not become congested from overexertion. As in Belladonna, Lycopodium has sudden vascular reactions such as hot flushes and local congestions.

Like Arsenicum and Rhus Tox., Lycopodium is restless at night and will get up to try and relieve his pains with movement, but in contrast to the former remedies, Lycopodium is worse before midnight and better at dawn.

As in Phosphorus, Arsenicum, Naja and Picricum Acidum, Lycopodium patients have the sensation of two hot coals in the middle of the back, between the scapulae.

Mental Symptoms

The mental symptoms accompany digestive problems. Patients will repeatedly state that when their digestion is bad, their moods change for the worse.

Worn down by worries, disappointments and vexations, they will often feel they are on the verge of a mental breakdown. They consider themselves to be highly-strung and sometimes even stop working to have a good rest. But these breaks do nothing to relieve these profoundly and chronically ill patients, whose symptoms are almost always triggered by fear, vexation, frustration, anxiety or disgust.

The Lycopodium depression is characterised by a marked failing of the memory and intellect. These patients are generally intelligent and well educated, and any noticeable decrease of mental faculties causes profound sadness and lack of self-confidence. Depression produces torpidity and the inability to carry out everyday tasks. As in Lachesis, the mental symptoms are aggravated on waking in the morning. Life feels like an intolerable burden; they feel utterly fed up and incapable of assuming any responsibilities whatsoever. Moodiness and general discontent upset family life. Lycopodium children awaken anxiously from nightmares, sit up in bed, fail to recognise their family and see ghosts with their eyes open until they fall asleep again, only to wake up in the morning feeling irritable and sluggish.

Lycopodium patients are incapable of focusing their attention; their thoughts escape them, they make mistakes when talking or writing, use the wrong words to express themselves, grope for the right words, omit words or letters when writing and may even forget the meaning of certain words. However, when they are excited because the matter at hand is important or when they choose to exert their willpower, the intellect can be surprisingly agile and efficient.

The decline in mental faculties makes Lycopodium patients feel inferior, sad, shy, reserved and cowardly; they tend to avoid people, meetings and public appearances.

They have a fear of failure, of being unable to carry on a conversation, and of revealing themselves in front of strangers. Lycopodium patients dislike being approached by new people and are intolerant of anyone who is not family or intimate friend. A keynote symptom is the fear of being alone, like Phosphorus, Arsenicum and Argentum Nitricum. As in Natrum Carbonicum, Aurum, Platinum and Pulsatilla, Lycopodium women fear men. Paradoxically, Lycopodium patients are averse to people but at the same time want to have their family in the next room. They are extremely emotional and will cry easily, even on happy occasions such as receiving a gift, being thanked for a favour or meeting a friend. Like Phosphorus, Anacardium, Natrum Muriaticum and Platinum, they laugh at serious matters.

Lycopodium has muscle spasms such as the sensation of a ball in the oesophagus, as found also in Ignatia, Lachesis and Pulsatilla, among others. Lycopodium's depression and melancholy may either lead to suicide or a state of utter indifference to everything, including family and children. It is useful in acute cases such as typhoid where there is the closed mouth, hanging jaw and half-closed eyes also seen in Opium, Muriaticum Acidum, Rhus Tox. and Causticum.

Mental depression is accompanied by fear, apprehension, sadness and irritability, impatience, discontent and oversensitivity. Lycopodium patients subconsciously try to cover up their lack of self-esteem with arrogance and intolerance.

There is an oversensitivity to noise, smells, pressure, and physical contact. Lycopodium is just as intolerant of contradiction, haughty and domineering, as Platinum or Sulphur. In acute conditions they complain about everything, greatly exaggerating their troubles and losing control as violently as Platinum, or as abusively as Anacardium or Iodum.

As in Aurum, Ignatia, Nux Vomica and Sulphur, Lycopodium is fond of arguing and fighting; but while in these other remedies violence is short-lived, in Lycopodium there is a more brooding anger. Lycopodium is one of the classic personality types in homoeopathy, the miserly, bad-tempered, dyspeptic misanthropist, just as Sulphur is the grimy, ragged, pretentious philosopher and Arsenicum is the thin, agitated, demanding, fastidious old man.

Synthesis

Lycopodium patients tend to be depressed; their weakened memory and intellect give rise to a lack of self-confidence, as well as fear of failure, apprehension, aversion to work, sadness, shyness, despondency and bad temper. Lycopodium's chronic kidney and liver deficiency causes the organism to retain metabolic toxins in the nervous, circulatory, skeletal systems and skin, as illustrated in the table opposite:

Nervous System	Emaciation Nervous debility Excitability Irritability	
Skeletal System	Muscles	Twitchings Sudden starts Paralysis
	Joints	Gout (tophus) Rigid, painful; modalities similar to Rhus Tox.
	Bones	Softening and caries
Circulatory System	Enlargement of the heart Arterial and circulatory disturbances, hot flushes Venous stasis, ascites, oedema, varicose veins	
Skin	Herpes Eczema Eruptions Ulcers Boils Anthrax Suppurations	

Rubrics and Related Remedies

Note: The author here has created a number of new rubrics and has added to existing rubrics.

Apprehension in stomach: Mezereum, Aurum, Cannabis Sativa, Digitalis Purpurea, Kali Carbonicum, Lycopodium, Phosphorus, Thuja. Anxious about being gravely ill.
Anticipation, want of self-confidence.
Desires to be alone, but wants to feel that people are at home or near. Afraid of being alone.
Fear in a crowd: Lycopodium, Pulsatilla, Rhus Tox.; in a warm room: Lycopodium, Pulsatilla, Sulphur, Iodum.

Fears people: Hyoscyamus, Lycopodium, Natrum Carbonicum, Rhus Tox.

Misanthropic.

Indifference towards his children.

Fear of others approaching him: Arnica, Ambra Grisea, Belladonna, Cuprum Metallicum, Ignatia, Lycopodium, Stramonium, Thuja.

Aversion to homoeopathy: Causticum, Hepar Sulphuris, Lycopodium, Nitricum Acidum, Nux Vomica, Sepia.

Aversion to opposite sex.

Sadness with mental confusion, tearful, feels wretched.

Spiritual depression, despairing, despondent, hypochondriac.

Sad when hearing music far away.

Melancholy. Fed up with life. Worse mornings.

Taciturn.

Sensitive. Cries when being thanked.

Fear of the dark, of going to bed at night.

Rude. Insolent.

Irritable, violent, bad-tempered. Intolerant of contradiction: Aurum, Ignatia, Lycopodium, Sepia. Easily roused to anger, annoyed by the slightest trifles.

Contradictory, reproaches others, argumentative, abusive. Bad temper on rising and in the morning generally; bad temper at dusk.

Irritability and bad temper before menses.

Cursing, swearing: Anacardium, Nitricum Acidum, Arsenicum, Hyoscyamus, Lilium Tigrinum, Lycopodium, Nux Vomica, Tuberculinum.

Discontented, bad-tempered, impatient, indifferent, apathetic children. Children who do not play.

Disobedience: Tarentula Hispanica, Lycopodium, China Officinalis, Ammonium Carbonicum.

Ailments from fright, rage, mortification or vexation.

Very sensitive to pain; pains exasperate: Chamomilla.

Concentration difficult.

Gropes for the right words with which to express thoughts.

When writing, omits and adds on letters.

Makes mistakes with words and syllables. Uses the wrong words.

Clever when rationalising about abstract topics, but confused about practical affairs of everyday life.

Very weak memory. Forgets the meaning of words or the use of letters.

Confusion and vertigo on getting up in the morning.

Conscientious about trifles: Ignatia, Silica, Arsenicum, Baryta Carbonica, Lycopodium, Natrum Carbonicum, Nux Vomica, Stramonium,

Lycopodium

Sulphur, Thuja.

Fastidious: Lycopodium, Staphysagria, Sulphur.

Cowardice: Gelsemium, Lycopodium.

Dictatorial: Camphora Officinarum, Lycopodium, Mercurius Vivus.

Presumptuous, imperious, domineering. Grumpy, grumbling.

Haughty: Lycopodium, Platinum, Sulphur, Veratrum Album, Causticum, Lachesis, Palladium, Staphysagria.

Egotism: Platinum, Lycopodium, Calcarea Carbonica, Palladium, Silica, Sulphur.

Envy: Pulsatilla, Staphysagria, Lycopodium.

Timidity, feels inferior, indecisive. Lacks faith in himself, as well as in friends, physician and remedies. Feels incompetent. Like Silica, avoids appearing in public, public gatherings, meetings, people in general, even his own children. Silent and taciturn. Does not want to talk, desires to be left alone in his room but needs to have someone near. Because intellectual contact with people is difficult due to mental debility, Lycopodium retreats into a shell, feigning indifference, disaffection and resignation to his lot. Sad, disheartened and easily moved to tears upon receiving a friend or when thanked for a service rendered or the least trifle.

Wakes in the morning dejected, fed up with life, despairing and often feeling as if there were a hand grasping the liver and other internal organs.

Lycopodium tries to cover up his physical weakness by assuming imperious, domineering and dictatorial airs and by acting presumptuously, with arrogance and haughtiness.

His impotence masquerades as distrust, malice, intolerance and offensive and quarrelsome behaviour. His oversensitivity makes him start at the sound of a ringing telephone or the slightest noise. Lycopodium and Gelsemium are the most cowardly of all the remedies in the materia medica; the former has the pride and insolence of Platinum, Veratrum Album and to a certain extent Sulphur.

Lycopodium speaks in a commanding, arrogant, bombastic manner and his sarcastic jokes are a defence mechanism for his innermost feelings of inferiority and pent-up aggression.

Chapter 25

Mercurius Solubilis
(1955)

Mercurius Solubilis is a precipitate of nitric acid; Mercurius Vivus is a trituration of pure quicksilver.

As mercury is not naturally present in the human organism, there is no mercury metabolism to compare with that of calcium, phosphorus, potassium or sodium. Nevertheless, mercury has the power to combine with most metals and metalloids – especially sulphur – and with the organism's ions, to disturb the metabolism's dynamic equilibrium.

Mercury reproduces the syphilitic symptom picture so faithfully that its remedial action has often been confused with syphilis. And when syphilitic mercury is combined with psoric sulphur, the result is the tubercular diathesis.

When mercury combines with potassium, sodium and chlorine it has a tremendous impact on the water metabolism. In cases of mercury poisoning, the kidneys are badly affected as they regulate water metabolism. This can be observed in nephritis cases where no urine is passed or in the remedial action of mercury-based diuretics.

Mercurius Solubilis is a syphilitic, scrofulous and lymphatic remedy. Mercurius patients have pale, earthy, bloated, swollen faces; red eyelids; cracked, dry lips; flaccid, cold, damp, clammy skin; foul, oily perspiration; and halitosis. The body exudes a most offensive odour.

Common symptoms are:

1) Marked sensitivity to both heat and cold, as if the organism itself were a thermometer.
2) Exacerbation of all symptoms at night, as in syphilis.
3) Profuse perspiration which brings no relief and generally worsens symptoms.
4) Fetid, mercurial odour from the breath, perspiration, excreta and suppurations.
5) Trembling of the fingers, as seen in Parkinson's disease, multiple sclerosis and general paralysis.

On the mental level Mercurius is rather feeble-minded, extremely restless, hurried in speech and too shy and embarrassed to answer questions. As in syphilis, Mercurius may damage the cerebral cortex and affect the intellect, leading to dullness, slowness and an immature, regressive personality. They feel insecure and out of control, anxious, apprehensive and uneasy. There is an overwhelming urge to kill or to commit suicide at the sight of a cutting instrument. Mercurius patients feel overwhelmed by their impulses and wish to escape from themselves, as if guilty of a crime. Unaware that the cause of the anxiety and fear is the enemy within, these patients look on everyone around them as their enemy. They fear being alone and believe they will lose their reason. They have a violent desire to kill the person who contradicts them and desire only to escape, even from time itself, which seems to pass very slowly.

The anxiety, fear and general restlessness become worse as night progresses, from 8.p.m. until the following morning.

Remedies that share a similar mental symptom picture are Aurum, Arsenicum, Hepar Sulphuris, Iodum, Nux Vomica and Platinum. As in Aurum, an antidote to Mercurius, they are full of self-reproach and guilty consciences. While Aurum thinks of suicide as a way to atone for guilt, Mercurius fears suicide and thinks only of escaping. The determinative symptom of Mercurius is the wish to kill whoever contradicts them and the person whom they love the most.

Arsenicum is so anxious and restless that he will jump out of bed after midnight, wishing to die. His impulses to kill are held in check by a great anxiety of conscience, as if the crime had actually been committed. There is much restlessness, with physical prostration.

Hepar Sulphuris is an aggressive remedy that flies into violent homicidal rages at the slightest provocation. The children never laugh or play, and have repulsive, destructive personalities. The adults are malevolent, potential criminals. with no moral conscience, as opposed to Aurum's tendency for self-reproach and inhibitions.

Iodum has an intense, feverish restlessness and anxiety that only lessens when eating. When forced to stay still, Iodum has manic impulses to kill, break things or commit other violent acts.

Nux Vomica is the typical stressed workaholic with unhealthy living habits. The mental and physical exhaustion may lead to either murder or suicide, or both.

Platinum expresses his irritability with insulting language, alternating between raging tears and convulsive laughter and taking pleasure in being cruel, sarcastic and destructive.

He is cold and arrogant and believes his disdainful judgments to be correct and that everyone else is small and inferior, both physically and morally. When Platinum comes face to face with his conscience he becomes profoundly depressed to the point of suicide, although his fear of death prevents him from taking his own life. However, the arrogance of Platinum is always evident, even in the midst of his darkest despair.

Platinum women are subject to bouts of hysterical tears and convulsive sarcastic laughter, and the physical symptoms alternate with the mental symptoms. They are cold, abusive and haughty, and despite their great sexual excitability and erotic dreams, reject their husbands. Platinum's mental trilogy is cruelty, pride and voluptuousness.

Argentum Nitricum, Medorrhinum, Nux Vomica and Mercurius are hurried and feel that time passes too slowly. Lilium Tigrinum, Natrum Muriaticum, Sulphur, Sulphuricum Acidum and Tarentula are agitated but do not feel that time passes slowly. On the other hand, Cannabis Indica, Glonoine and Nux Moschata are not agitated but do feel as if time passed by very slowly. Cannabis Indica has an altered notion of space and time; a few metres seem like a long distance; a few minutes like hours, as opposed to Cocculus, for whom time passes quickly.

Mercurius suffers from bad headaches at night. The forehead feels tight, as if gripped by a tight bandage with deep, tearing, sharp, burning pains. Whereas Syphilinum headaches are linear, Mercurius headaches are constrictive. The following morning there is a dizzy, confused, heavy feeling in the head. The head feels full, congested, apoplectic and about to burst; always worse by both heat and cold.

Mercurius patients may suffer from syphilitic, rheumatic or catarrhal headaches; worse by suppression of discharges such as foot-sweat, catarrh, rhinitis, otorrhoea and leucorrhoea; better for discharges.

The cranium is painful to the touch, with sensitive exostosis. The scalp feels taut and constricted. A lot of hair falls out at the temples.

As in Calcarea Carbonica, Calcarea Phosphorica, Lycopodium, Sepia and Sulphur, Mercurius children have large hydrocephalic heads, Olympian foreheads, broad fontanelles, open sutures and cold, profuse, oily perspiration during sleep, soaking the pillow at night. Mercurius children may also have rickets, eczema and impetigo with dry, fetid yellow crusts.

The mucous membranes of the body orifices have copious, runny, irritating and fetid catarrh and greenish-yellow suppurations and ulcerations.

Chronic syphilitic ophthalmia is frequently seen in Mercurius. Lacrimation is copious and excoriating. There is runny, acrid suppuration, sharp pains in the eye sockets and temples, and a marked sensitivity to light. Retinitis, choroiditis, iriditis, pustular and parenchymatous keratitis, pustular conjunctivitis and erysipelatoid blepharitis are also characteristic of this remedy. All symptoms are worse at night and from heat.

As in Apis, Mercurius suffers from chronic suppurating otitis with thick, offensive discharges; stabbing, piercing pains in the ears, worse at night. Polyps and furuncles develop in the auditory canal.

As in Arsenicum Album and Iodatum, Mercurius has acute, feverish coryza. There is much sneezing and profuse, corrosive, foul-smelling discharges. Itchy nose, crusts; epistaxis with catarrh and flu symptoms. Much congestion, especially of the upper mucous membranes, including the postnasal sinuses. Muscular fatigue, sour, profuse perspiration at night which does not bring relief. Intolerance of cold and heat.

Mercurius also has chronic rhinitis with foul-smelling, greenish-yellow excoriating and ulcerative discharges and inflammation of the nasal bones, which Syphilinum corrodes and destroys. Nocturnal epistaxis is a common feature.

This remedy exerts a deep remedial action on the two extremes of the digestive tract – that is, the mouth and pharynx and the rectum and anus. Stomatitis with putrid-smelling breath is typical of Mercurius and of the syphilitic and tubercular miasms.

The tongue is swollen, flabby, yellow, and teeth-indented. There is much trembling in the tongue, which makes speech difficult. There is copious, viscous, frothy, fetid salivation with a metallic taste at night. A disturbed water metabolism causes intense thirst despite profuse salivation.

There is gum disease, spongy, receding gums with easy bleeding; with small aphthae and a reddish-violet border around the teeth. Cavities develop easily, and the teeth are often dirty grey or even black and loose in their sockets.

In an acute symptom picture, the mucous membranes of the throat and upper respiratory tract turn dark red, and in spite of the profuse salivation feel dry and burning. Swallowing is painful, and the pain extends to the ears.

Ulcers and thrush develop with grey membranous tissue. Enlarged tonsils may suppurate or be covered with membranous tissue. The uvula and fauces are swollen. There is much foul-smelling salivation, dry thirst, fever and pains which extend to the ears upon swallowing.

In diphtheria cases, Mercurius Cyanatus is a much better simillimum than Mercurius Solubilis, whereas cases of dysentery will respond to Mercurius Solubilis. Frothy, offensive, bloody, irritating stools. As in

Plumbum and Cuprum, Mercurius has frequent, ineffectual urgings produced by spasms of the colon and may lead to a prolapsed rectum. The rectum feels as if some stool remains.

There is both polyuria and dysuria. Tenesmus is common with only a little urine passed at a time, sudden, frequent urges to urinate, and incontinence. Urine burns as it is being expelled, has much sediment and may be murky, mahogany-coloured, milky-white, albuminous or bloody. Albuminous nephritis or uraemia with anuria may develop.

The male sexual organs have abnormal sensitivity with frequent erections, and ejaculations which may be bloody. Masturbation in male infants, who pull on their prepuce all night.

The remedy can also have impotence with a cold and flaccid penis. The prepuce has inflammation, ulcers and offensive pus. The testicles are inflamed and feel heavy.

There is profuse perspiration around the genitals with excoriations in the folds of the groin and scrotum.

The female has metrorrhagia with thick blood clots and intense, menstrual cramps. Scanty menses for several months. Hot flushes before and during periods with intense, dry heat and pelvic congestion.

Profuse, excoriating, acid, corrosive and greenish leucorrhoea with much itching in the genital area, which burns on scratching; better by washing with cold water.

Sterility with profuse menstruation, or becomes easily pregnant.

Painful nodules and adenomas on the breasts during menstrual periods.

Secretion of milk instead of menstrual periods. Milk on little girl's nipples.

Excoriation of the nipples after childbirth; the infant rejects the mother's breast.

Rheumatic, lacerating, tearing pains in the back and legs, aggravated at night by the heat of the bed and by perspiration. Trembling limbs, especially the hands. Paralysis agitans, such as in Parkinson's disease. Multiple sclerosis, general paralysis. Essential tremor.

Paralytic weakness of the lower limbs, feeling hot inside, yet skin feels cold. Cramps and contractions in the calves and toes.

The skin is pale and yellowish, with profuse, clammy, offensive perspiration at night that stains the clothes and does not relieve the patient.

As in syphilis, copper-hued stains develop on the skin that turn purple with the cold.

Pustule-like eruptions with nocturnal itch and the sensation of flea-bites, worse by the heat of the bed.

Irregularly shaped skin ulcers where the skin comes in contact with the bones, such as the crown of the tibia. Ulcers are irregularly shaped with undefined borders and have purulent, fetid, corrosive secretions. In the acute stage, Mercurius has alternating chills and heat. The first chills often happen at night, followed by heat and perspiration which does not relieve the patient.

Mental Symptoms

Feeble-minded, diminished intellectual powers, poor memory. Idiocy, smiles stupidly. Cries constantly with no apparent cause. Great sadness. Does not understand; speaks incoherently. Absent-minded, distracted. Embarrassed, perplexed, upset, confused.
Dull, obtuse, with a great inclination to sleep.
Mischievous, destructive, perverse, malevolent, gossipy, meddler.
Delirium with muttering; delirium tremens.
Desire to kill or to commit suicide. Worse during menstrual periods.
Ideas of suicide at the sight of cutting instruments or an open window.
Fears making a mistake and thereupon having to kill himself.
Desire to kill the person that contradicts him.
Anxiety and restlessness, constantly shifts position. Fear of insanity. Hot flushes and perspiration, does not know what to do, apprehensive, full of fears. Many imaginary fears. Worse at night and at dusk. Thoughts of suicide, wishes to die, believes he is becoming insane. Great indifference towards people he has loved before. Cries involuntarily, which brings relief.
Hysteria. Hypochondria. Hysterical melancholy with an inclination to kill.
Loathing of life.
State of melancholy with indescribable depression. Restless anxiety, as if an illness or an evil were to befall him. Worse at night, with precordial anxiety, sweating palms and hot flushes in the face. Disgusted with himself, lacks the courage to live; suspects everyone; considers everyone his enemy. Grief with fear at nightfall. Feels as if head were about to burst.
Anxiety of conscience, as if guilty of a crime. Great restlessness, does not want to eat, even though when he does so it is with great appetite. Ideas impinge upon the mind, one after the other. Tendency to pull the nose when walking.
Desire to travel, to go abroad. Nocturnal anxiety with perspiration. Desire to escape.

Restlessness, worse at night. Does not remain in the same position for a single moment. Cannot rest anywhere, constantly anxious.
Bad effects of frights which leave him in a state of great anxiety.
Effects of mortification, insults, selfishness.
Hurried and rapid talking. Feels as if time passes very slowly.

Head

The whole head is very sensitive and painful to the touch. Head feels very big.
Congestion of the head, sensation of fullness, as if it were about to burst.
Feels as if head were in a band or in a vice.

Eyes

Blurred vision, sees sparks, visions of insects, sensitive to light, lacrimation, suppuration, inflamed eyelids.

Nose

Nosebleeds during sleep, feels as if weight were hanging from the nose.
Profuse, foul-smelling coryza with pain in the bones. Feels as if cold water were oozing out of the ears.

Mouth

Cracks in the corner of the mouth. Feels as if teeth were becoming loose. Swollen tongue. Thrush. Sharp pains in teeth at night with chills. Swollen gums which separate from the teeth. Gums bleed at slightest contact and hurt when chewing. Copious salivation, foul breath, pale white tongue with imprint of teeth, with yellowish-white gastric sordes. Bad breath which impregnates the room.
Salivary glands swollen and painful; copious salivation.
Sweetish taste in the mouth. Salty taste on the lips or tongue. Dry throat, intense thirst.

Urinary System

Burning sensation in the urethra, constant desire to urinate. Profuse urination voiding more than he has drunk.

Skin

Copious perspiration; worse by perspiration.
Large, bleeding ulcers, painful to the touch. Tendency to develop suppurations and ulcers.

Stool

Exhausted after defecating.

Extremities

Pains in the bones, especially in those covered by thin skin, such as the tibia, worse at night, worse by the heat of the bed, with profuse discharges, worse by perspiration.

General Symptoms

Offensive-smelling body.
Sensitive to both heat and cold.
Acrid, excoriating, greenish discharges.
Chilly, weak, trembling with fear.

Chapter 26

Natrum Muriaticum
(1956)

Together with five of his provers, Hahnemann introduced and experimented with Natrum Muriaticum. Later on, Austrian physicians performed additional provings. Regarding salt, Hahnemann states in *The Chronic Diseases* that:

> If, furthermore, as experience teaches, all substances that should have the power of healing diseases must, on the other hand, be able to affect injuriously the state of healthy men, it would be hard to see how all nations on earth, even those only half-civilized, should have daily used salt in not inconsiderable quantities, for so many thousands of years, without experiencing any deleterious effects on the human health ...

> If we then assume that common salt in its natural condition, shows no injurious effects on the human health, when used daily in moderate quantity, we ought not to expect from it any curative effects in diseases. Nevertheless, the greatest medicinal virtues lie hidden within it.

> If there is then any proof convincing even the most dim-sighted, that the preparation of drugs, peculiar to Homoeopathy, opens, as it were, a new world of forces, which hitherto have lain hidden by nature, this proof is surely afforded by the transformation of common salt, so indifferent in its crude state, into a heroic and mighty medicine, which, after such preparation, can only be given to patients with the greatest care. What an incredible and yet actual transformation! Apparently a new creation!

Natrum Muriaticum is a tubercular remedy that is often emaciated, dehydrated, devitalised, weak and exhausted, and suffers from Stiller's asthenia. There is a combination of deep sadness, melancholy, irritability and palpitations.

As sodium chloride is an indispensable element for organic hydration and the fixation of mineral salts, Natrum Muriaticum patients have deeply disturbed mineral metabolisms; as all biological processes take place in a saline medium, it is more than likely that a sodium chloride imbalance will occur some time in the life of every human organism. Consequently, Natrum Muriaticum is a remedy that is often indicated – especially when the body's requirements for mineral salts are higher, as in childhood, puberty and adolescence, tuberculous primary infections, pregnancy and old age.

Sad, indifferent, joyless and easily offended by the most harmless joke, Natrum Muriaticum is intolerant of contradiction. He is annoyed by the slightest trifles, easily roused to unreasonable anger and vehemence.

Once Natrum Muriaticum has been prescribed, the patient will feel calm, mellow, content, hopeful and free from anxiety. His anxiety, in fact, stems from pent-up anger. No matter what the illness, if a patient is constitutionally Natrum Muriaticum and his resentment is not cured, either it is not the right remedy or something is interfering with its remedial action.

To understand this basic component of Natrum Muriaticum, it is necessary to understand aggression.

Resentment stems from pent-up aggression, a basic, primary instinct of self-preservation, along with the need for self-affirmation and domination. A patient's frustration may be caused by events in his life, too many inhibitions or prohibitions in his upbringing, or an innate weakness. Thus, the impoverished ego is incapable of withstanding small frustrations which would be considered normal and insignificant by stronger constitutions.

Hereditary influence manifests itself when given the appropriate environmental conditions. However, as in all of life's circumstances, the response to emotional frustrations depends upon the individual's innate predisposition.

Calcarea Carbonica will respond with apathetic fear; Silica with stubborn bashfulness; Sulphur with irritable selfishness; Pulsatilla with tearfulness and a need for dependency; Platinum with a disdainful attitude; Lycopodium with pride; Hepar Sulphuris with ferocious irritability; Arsenicum with anxiety and restlessness; Aurum with anxiety of conscience; Phosphorus with intensified fear; Natrum Muriaticum with resentment.

Natrum Muriaticum patients are weak, insecure, lacking in courage. They become irritated by frustration but dare not express their anger, and thus turn it against themselves, bringing on profound melancholy, sadness, dejection and anxious despair with palpitations. These are undoubtedly resentful patients who dwell on thoughts about the injuries they have received or wished upon others, and become depressed to the point of not finding pleasure in anything.

They bury themselves in sad, depressing thoughts, dwell on unpleasant events from the past, weep against their will and think of what will become of them. They believe that others pity them, and are aggravated by any attempt at consolation.

Weeping is a way of releasing their pent-up aggression because, as in Staphysagria, they cannot express rage.

They are unable to assert themselves or exercise their will, and feel sad, hopeless, weak, indifferent, disgusted with their work, easily distracted and unable to perform mental work. Lack of coordination between the nervous and motor systems, clumsiness and dropping things may also be present.

However, there are times when Natrum Muriaticum suddenly becomes very cheerful, wants to sing and dance, and with eyes filled with tears will burst into hysterical, uncontrollable laughter, another way of releasing pent-up rage. This is not distinctively characteristic of the remedy, as it is in Pulsatilla. Natrum Muriaticum leans more towards obsessive neurosis than hysteria.

During sleep, when subconscious activity is free from the pressure of conscious censorship, Natrum Muriaticum patients have terrible nightmares. Vivid dreams of burglars (their own hostile drives) are common. When awake, they make sure the burglars are really not there. They cry in their sleep, and wake up feeling dull, listless and with pains around the waist.

Now, we must take care to distinguish Natrum Muriaticum from the other sad remedies of the materia medica. Natrum Muriaticum is resentful, silent, melancholy and full of self-pity. Aurum has anxiety of conscience, self-blame and suicidal thoughts; Causticum craves sympathy and protection, but without resentment; apathetic Conium is calm and apathetic with excitability or anxiety; Kali Phosphoricum has meekness, mental prostration, is oversensitive to noise, easily startled and hypochondriac; fickle, whimsical Pulsatilla is easily influenced and controlled; Plumbum is mentally paralysed; Psorinum may feel desperately anxious about salvation and a deep-seated, pessimistic fear of everything; finally, Sepia impassively seeks solitude without consolation, as Natrum Muriaticum does, but with indifference.

As we have seen, a remedy's characteristic symptom picture is made up of subjective symptoms and modalities which reveal a dynamic tendency to generate certain pathological processes. Although we have not yet been able to understand the pathogenesis of the causal relationship involved, the objective and pathological signs which complete the image are gathered from repeated clinical observations and link a specific pathology to a specific dynamic disturbance. Because the true determinative symptoms of a remedy do not follow the usual logic of physiopathology, Hahnemann called them strange, rare and peculiar symptoms.

Natrum Muriaticum patients lack vital heat and at the same time are prone to heat exhaustion, especially in the summer sun. There is an increased appetite, with emaciation of the upper half of their bodies, anxiety with palpitations, extreme thirst, desire for salty and bitter foods and beer, aversion to bread, chronic catarrh of the nose and throat like egg-white, stuffy nose, herpes on the lips and around the mouth, and throbbing headaches with vertigo. They are worse on awakening or at 10 a.m. and often have an oily face as in Thuja, Plumbum and Selenium. Natrum Muriaticum women feel worse during menstrual periods, and irritable before them.

Three of the above symptoms along with the mental syndrome, which of course always takes precedence, are enough to characterise the essence of Natrum Muriaticum.

They are joyless, pessimistic people with an inferiority complex, either emotionally dependent on the mother or proud or indifferent, as in Phosphorus or Sepia.

Natrum Muriaticum is a tubercular remedy, and mental symptoms may be less significant in a comparative study with Tuberculinum. The latter has fearful anxiety, extreme irritability with angry outbursts and profound depression.

Tuberculinum and Natrum Muriaticum can be differentiated by their general symptoms. Tuberculinum is changeable, restless, always wishing to move house, go travelling and change his surroundings; he feels well one day; poorly the next; catches cold easily, with no apparent cause, and there is usually a history of tuberculosis in the family with infarcted ganglions, enlarged tonsils, eczema, a tendency to perspire and lose weight. Tuberculinum is chilly and needs cold air.

These symptoms are similar to Natrum Muriaticum, but can define a case as such only after Tuberculinum has acted.

Natrum Muriaticum patients are neurotics. The frustrations they have suffered have exacerbated their hatred and unleashed a morbid process that may be understood by examining the patient's constitution.

These days all biological processes of adaptation are studied in terms of reactivity. Neurosis is now considered along the same lines as hypersensitivity or allergy. It is precisely this capacity for reaction that lays the foundation for psora – mankind's fundamental disease, according to Hahnemann.

Whether due to susceptibility, hypersensitivity or allergy, psora is the capacity to react, not only to physical conditions such as climate, temperature, food and infections, but also to emotional provocation, such as criticism, aggression, hate, humiliation, vexation, lack of affection, frustration and so on. The individual is predisposed to react in specific ways to these challenges that may be triggered by frustrating or repressive childhood experiences.

The underlying cause of the patient's neurotic constitution is to be found in his personal history and family background.

Neurosis and organic disease must be considered as ways in which the individual's personality reacts to the disturbance, rather than as diseases as such. This disturbance expresses itself as either a mental or physical ailment and reflects the individual's reaction to the process of adaptation to the outer world.

In early childhood, the organism throws up a series of cleansing diseases such as nettle rash, prurigo, eczema, measles and whooping cough (psoric), scarlet fever (syphilitic) and colds (sycotic).

Organic disease is the result of the repression of morbid energy and the frustrations that the vital force tries ineffectually to release, whether on the mental or the physical level.

A patient's life history is a record of the suppressions and frustrations he has suffered in trying to adapt as his personality evolves.

Emotional frustration, then, is a form of suppression which interferes with the psychological and hormonal development of the human being in the first stages of infancy. To adapt successfully to life, the child needs love and emotional security. He needs to expand to express himself and become a mature responsible adult. He must overcome fear and anxiety and struggle to gain a sense of self-worth, to maintain the empowering belief that he is capable, useful, self-assertive and self-sufficient. This instinctive need for self-assertion, power, success or superiority, is at the bottom of all basic human conflicts and all disease.

To feel emotionally secure the child needs to be understood in terms of his vital need for self-sufficiency and self-esteem. Children who have not received this understanding are likely to suffer frustrations that will affect their emotional and physical development towards maturity, self-sufficiency and freedom.

The emotional frustration of which we speak here is not the over-protecting love of the parents, but the breakdown of the psychological support that the child needs to develop and adapt to life.

The yearning for love is the yearning for parental security that helps the child to become self-supportive, to respond appropriately and freely to life's demands, to master reality and to conquer freedom.

When questioned, resentful patients will rarely complain that their parents did not love them, but rather that they did not understand them. This is a blatant appeal to external identification with their own need to love, to succeed, to express and assert themselves.

Admirable parents are those who help their children succeed, not by spoiling and overprotecting them, but by understanding them and, through their own example, aiding the natural law of evolution towards autonomy, towards the freedom which is every person's instinctive goal. In order to evolve towards freedom, the child requires security and love, not the severing of his potential. A lack of love will lead to frustration, insecurity and fear and an inability to respond with maturity to the demands of life.

Constitutional

Anaemia, blood; emaciation; nutrition; dehydration.

Mental Symptoms

Sensitive, emotional, always on the verge of tears. Introverted. (Extro-verted, Phosphorus.)

Discontent, dissatisfied with everything. Bumbling when talking or thinking.

Torments himself; recalling insults, offences, betrayals in love.

Feels extremely unfairly treated and mortified.

Does not want to be pitied; irritable; rejects all consolation.

Better alone. Hides tears for fear of being pitied or consoled. Sad when consoled. As in Ignatia, cannot weep. (Sepia prefers to be alone outside of her house.)

Averse to company, noise and consolation. Malicious; malevolent: Nux Vomica, Hepar Sulphuris, Nitricum Acidum.

As opposed to Pulsatilla, who wants pity, Natrum Muriaticum feels inferior and weeps when others look at or thank him. Weeps over past events.

Rancorous, vindictive, thirsts for revenge. Anger from fright, vexation or past mortification.

Trembling after a fright.

Paralysis after a fit of anger, passion or manic depression.

Falls in love with an inappropriate person and is gripped by an uncontrollable passion. Hysterical young women with impossible loves.

Ailments from disappointed love: Ignatia, Natrum Muriaticum, Phosphoricum Acidum.

Agitation, anxious haste with palpitations; always hurried.

Hysterical fits of laughter with tears as if he had been weeping.

Indifferent; hypochondriac; taciturn. Tired of life: Phosphorus.

Does not tolerate the presence of others while urinating (Ambra Grisea while defecating).

Misanthropy. Wishes to be alone in order to weep or masturbate.

As in Phosphorus, fears something will happen; anxious about the future.

Fears insanity, burglars, storms.

Irritable; impatient. Bad-tempered when constipated and better when bowels are relieved.

Hysterical alternating between great sadness and euphoria.

Feels pursued.

As in Sepia, aversion to men and sexual intercourse.

During pregnancy, fears that the child will be monstrously deformed.

Annoyed by trifles.

Indifferent.

Feels mentally sluggish, empty-headed.

Head

As in Belladonna, throbbing, oppressive pains as if the head were about to burst, but with anaemia.

Headaches preceded by visual disturbances; school headaches. Periodic migraine headaches.

Eyes

Twitching eyelids.

Mouth

Herpes on the lips, cracked lower lip.

Mapped, cracked tongue.

Stomach

Unquenchable thirst.

Craves salt. Averse to fat. Either craves bread or is averse to it.

Female

Scanty menses. Chlorosis. Anaemia.

Heart

Palpitations; rapid heartbeats with hypotension (anaemia). Palpitations are felt all over body and cause jerking. Intermittent heartbeats. Cold sensation in heart.

Skin

Eczematous eruption along the hair margin and nape of neck.
Eczema in folds of the skin.

Modalities

Worse from 9 to 10 a.m. Worse as sun travels its course. Worse by seashore.

Children

Children who look under the bed or inside the cupboard before going to bed at night.

As in Agaricus Muscarius and Baryta Carbonica, children who are late in learning to talk and, as in Calcarea Carbonica, late in learning to walk.

Thin, emaciated children, especially in the neck region. Dry, wrinkled skin.

Pale, yellowish, greasy face, with dry, cracked, blistered lips.

Acne-like eruptions on the skin.

Watery coryza that ulcerates and causes cracks.

Averse to fatty foods.

Better when eating little or not eating at all. As in Iodum, may have bulimia.

Cannot tolerate jokes. Children who are easily offended when they think they are being made fun of.

Mortification: exaggerated feeling of being treated unfairly, feels frustrated, cheated, ignored. Colocynthis, Ignatia, Lycopodium, Natrum Muriaticum, Palladium, Phosphoricum Acidum, Staphysagria, Argentum Nitricum, Aurum, Bryonia, Chamomilla, Pulsatilla, Sulphur.

Homesickness: Capsicum, Carbo Animalis, Phosphoricum Acidum, Aurum, Causticum, Ignatia, Kali Phosphoricum, Natrum Muriaticum, Silica, Staphysagria.

Hurry: Lilium Tigrinum, Medorrhinum, Mercurius, Natrum Muriaticum, Sulphur, Sulphuricum Acidum, Tarentula Hispanica.

Weeping when alone: Conium Maculatum, Natrum Muriaticum.

Dwells on past disagreeable occurrences: Natrum Muriaticum, Ambra Grisea, Chamomilla, China, Cocculus, Conium Maculatum, Platinum, Sepia, Sulphur.

Gum disease; (scorbutic) pyorrhoea: Natrum Muriaticum, Ammonium Carbonicum, Nux Vomica.

Emaciated children: Arsenicum Album, Arsenicum Iodatum, Calcarea Carbonica, Calcarea Phosphorica, Iodum, Natrum Muriaticum, Silica, Lycopodium, Phosphorus, Psorinum, Pulsatilla, Sepia, Sulphur.

Slow in learning to talk: Natrum Muriaticum, Agaricus Muscarius; Baryta Carbonica, Calcarea Phosphorica, Nux Moschata, Sanicula Aqua.

Hangnails: Natrum Muriaticum, Sulphur, Calcarea Carbonica, Lycopodium, Mercurius Solubilis, Rhus Tox., Silica, Stannum Metallicum, Thuja.

Chapter 27

Nitricum Acidum
(1955)

Nitricum Acidum has a long history of chronic ailments with emaciation. The pale, yellowish complexion is waxy with copper-coloured moles. The eyes are sunken and puffy, with a yellow areola. The lips and corners of the mouth are cracked and blistered. They are sad, anguished, desperate, misanthropic patients who often suffer from coryza, prolonged suppurations, ulcerations and diarrhoea.

They feel hopeless and forsaken and believe the whole world is against them. They reject people and are resentful, aggressive and anxious. Trapped by feelings of anguish and despair they both fear and long for death. They become gripped by fits of rage, trembling and hurling insults and curses at others. They permit no excuses or apologies and are completely unrepentant. They are cranky, irritable, dissatisfied with everything and everyone, including themselves. The mood alternates between raging anger, indifference and lethargy.

They are bitter, bad-tempered and resentful, prone to anger, stubbornness, indifference and insults. Symptoms may come on after the loss of a loved one or prolonged anxiety about the illness of someone dear to them.

They are unable to concentrate, their thoughts are scattered and any mental effort causes tiredness.

There is great physical weakness and trembling.
Lack of vital heat, very sensitive to cold, air currents and wind.
Muscular contractions in different parts of the body.
Pains that start and stop suddenly.
Excessive hunger with great debility and emaciation.

Physical symptoms of lesser importance are as follows:

Heat aggravates but hot applications ameliorate.
Milk and fatty foods aggravate.
Gnawing pains in the bones.
Pains feel like splinters or slivers of glass.

189

Strong, penetrating odour of the whole body and excreta.
Tendency to bleed easily; bright red blood.
Excoriations and cracks in all orifices.
Tendency to produce ulcers, fissures, cracks and fistulae.
Hardened ganglions and glands.
Purulent, greenish-yellow discharges from the mucous membranes.

Nitricum Acidum is an antisyphilitic, antisycotic and antipsoric remedy, similar to Thuja in its general and particular symptoms.

Chapter 28

Phosphorus
(1957)

The fourteen major components of the human organism are carbon, hydrogen, oxygen, nitrogen, sulphur, chlorine, potassium, sodium, calcium, magnesium, iron, silica, fluorine and phosphorus.

Phosphorus regulates the catabolic process and acts on the cell nuclei, nerve cells and visceral tissue. In toxic doses, Phosphorus speeds up combustion. An internal fire is lit, so to speak, accelerating all functions and exhausting reserves of vital energies.

Both current and constitutional symptom pictures must be studied in depth. Sometimes a current, acute symptom picture may call for a constitutional remedy; at other times it may not. When constitutional remedies are called for in an acute disease, the patient's excretory organs and structural pathology must be carefully assessed in order to avoid causing irreversible aggravations.

Remedies are divided into those which have a local, organic, superficial, short-range action and those which dynamically influence the innermost constitution. The first group of remedies, known as drainage remedies, generally cover the current symptom picture, but the second group are truly curative, even though it may not be possible to prescribe them immediately.

Although Phosphorus is basically a constitutional remedy it may also be prescribed for localised action in acute cases when indicated. Shortly after its discovery in 1673 by Henning Brand, an alchemist from Hamburg, phosphorus was used for medicinal purposes. Its main toxicological and therapeutic properties include heart, liver, respiratory and nervous affections and the well-known necrosis of the mandible observed in workers who handle phosphorus.

Its toxic action on tissues is characterised by destruction, caries and necrosis; it removes calcium from the bones, destroys the red blood cells and produces a fatty degeneration of the liver, kidneys, pancreas and muscles.

It is a highly reactive and oxidisable chemical, and thus a powerful reductant. It is present in every tissue in the form of phosphates and organic compounds, is an essential part of the cell nucleus, and plays an important role in nutrition and reproduction. It is found in the lecithin of the brain and nerves and affects them both. It contributes to the formation of diphosphoglyceric acid and causes haemorrhaging in red blood cells. A toxic dose of phosphorus brings on vomiting, diarrhoea, intense pains all over the body and bleeding from all orifices.

Thumbnail sketches of the most common constitutional remedies depict Sulphur as congested, ruddy-faced, self-obsessed and wilful; Lycopodium as sensitive, irritable, arrogant and prone to liver affections; Sepia as hypertense, with an outlook on life as black as the cuttlefish's cloud of ink; Natrum Muriaticum as sad, resentful, malnourished and dehydrated; Kali Carbonicum as oedematous, anaemic, fearful and easily startled; Iodum as thin, anxious and agitated, with infarcted glands and ganglia; Arsenicum as anxious and agitated, with burning pains and putrefaction; Pulsatilla as craving fresh air, shy, emotional and changeable; Calcarea Carbonica as apprehensive, slow and apathetic; and Phosphorus as oversensitive, extremely lethargic and prone to bleed easily.

Phosphorus patients tend to be tall, thin and emaciated due to their overactive metabolisms. They have the delicate, white, wax-like, transparent skin and long eyelashes of pretubercular patients. They tend to grow rapidly, have a long, thin thorax and a curved spine. Anaemia and a sanguine temperament are often present. They have keen senses, vivid perceptions and reactions, a tendency to bleed and bruise easily, and a marked oversensitivity with heat flushes, burning sensations and congestion.

Phosphorus is oversensitive to touch, odours, noises, and electrical changes in the atmosphere. He overreacts to minor difficulties with sudden fits of enthusiasm, aggression or weeping. The vitality is deeply deranged and prone to softening, atrophy and tissue damage, with eventual paralysis.

There are tremendous mood swings from agitation, anxiety, manic-depression, sexual arousal, anger and violence to apathy, indifference, prostration, deep depression, melancholy, trembling and paralysis. Indeed, the remedy is capable of complete self-annihilation.

Phosphorus is restless and fearful and cannot sit still for a single moment. When alone, at dusk, the fears, apprehensions, forebodings and restlessness are intensified. The fears, felt in the pit of the stomach, are of death, apoplexy or brain haemorrhage (a fear fed by the violent rushes of blood to the head), lightning and thunderstorms (causing palpitations, diarrhoea and trembling), water, insanity, suffocation and disease. There are also fears of unforeseen events, being alone, darkness, magic spells, burglars, ghosts, spirits, faces that peer out from corners and other imagined things. A piano being played will also bring on fear in Phosphorus.

The restlessness and fear may trigger fibrillar contractions, burning, tearing, and drawing pains, rigidity, trembling, numbness and tingling sensations which indicate spinal irritation. These symptoms are often followed by apathy, listlessness, lack of affection, indifference towards their own children, family and friends, hypochondria, deep sadness, inability to sustain mental effort, apprehension and a sinking sensation in the pit of the stomach. There may be paraplegia, hemiplegia, ataxia, unsteadiness and a fuzzy feeling on the soles of the feet. There may be progressive paralysis with insanity and delusions of grandeur.

Often, Phosphorus patients will have forebodings of terrible and imminent calamities that may even drive them to suicide. These fears are manifestations of the tubercular diathesis and syphilitic miasm. Psora provides the foundation for all disease, and psora and syphilis combine to form the tubercular diathesis. Psora represents the life instinct, hence the acute diseases and discharges produced by the vital force. Superimposed on psora is the death instinct which leads to tuberculosis or annihilation through insanity or suicide. All of Phosphorus's fears stem from a basic fear of his own destructive impulses. Phosphorus, so to speak, carries his own assassin within.

Suicide is murder of the self; the murderer is also the victim. Suicide may be brought about by a fatal destiny which subtly creates the appropriate circumstances for inevitable destruction.

Aurum's destructive tendencies manifest as aggression towards the self. Phosphorus is too fearful to commit suicide. However, there are many other forms of self-destruction, such as patients who avoid the cure they say they want, and patients who submit to mutilating operations to assuage their thirst for destruction or leave their own annihilation in the hands of destiny, so to speak.

Modern psychology maintains that there are both positive tendencies for growth, and negative tendencies of rejection, aggression and death. The destructive instinct accompanies all vital processes, both biological and psychological, and seeks to destroy that which stimulates the vital force; just as we break down the food we ingest in order to assimilate it, so we unconsciously create the circumstances of our own destiny.

The Phosphorus patient has a deep-seated fear of his aggressive impulses, producing a state of anxiety with agitation, constant restlessness and the whole gamut of fears. The syphilitic Aurum patient's response is an anxiety of conscience. Aurum patients are full of guilt, remorse, self-reproach and despair of salvation, and consider suicide as the only escape. Although generally too fearful to commit suicide, Phosphorus patients are nevertheless quite capable of carrying it out if they become desperate.

Arsenicum patients are capable of committing suicide because their fear of death is the destructiveness of their exhausted organisms. Psorinum patients are also capable of committing suicide because they despair of recovery and of salvation and feel unable to stem the tide of encroaching deterioration.

Phosphorus is easily roused and subject to uncontrollable sexual thoughts and erections. But at the same time, as Hahnemann pointed out, the vital force is wanting. The sexual instinct – the fullest expression of the life instinct – is so strongly linked to the death instinct, that the sexual act becomes dangerous and harmful to the subject, thus turning into a taboo.

One Phosphorus patient, a young man of twenty-three, admitted that he feared sexual intercourse. He had never had sex and was horrified at the thought of having to perform the sexual act. Convinced that his testicles were atrophied and feeling hopelessly impotent, when this young man was with his girlfriend, he was gripped by a terrible fear of causing her harm, of abusing her both physically and emotionally, even of destroying her life. He believed that suicide would be his only escape, but his intense fear of death held him back.

His other symptoms were: great excitement and restlessness; hot flushes which extended from his hands to his face; frequent washing of the hands which often felt hot and dry; congestive headaches improved by cold applications; burning thirst for cold water; large appetite with fainting and languor; acrocyanosis of the fingers and pains worse on the left side. He also bled quite easily; when shaving, he had to use a special pencil prepared with alum and blood ferment extract. Blood coagulation is severely impaired in Phosphorus; blood may ooze out of every orifice. Bleeding of the nose and lungs, urinating blood and blood in the sputum when cold are common occurrences, as well as purpuric spots; spontaneous bruises, petechias (in acute symptom pictures) and copious bleeding of small wounds.

This tendency to bleed easily is often seen with cardiovascular disease. Phosphorus has burning, tearing, drawing pains all over the body; burning sensations between the shoulderblades; burning sensations in specific points along the spinal column and running up the spinal column; blood rushing to the head; stuffy, throbbing headaches; hot flushes which radiate from the hands to the face and, as in Syphilinum, a frequent urge to wash the hands because they feel hot and dry.

The head and stomach symptoms are better by cold and are worse by heat, hot applications, sticking the hands in hot water and by eating hot food. However all other symptoms pertaining to the rest of the body are worse by cold and better by heat.

There is intense congestion with a general sensitivity to cold and gastric congestion, ameliorated by cold foods and cold drink, which may be vomited once it is warmed in the stomach. The lips, mouth and throat are very dry and there is a marked desire for ice cream, which soothes stomach pains.

Thirsty, congested and bleeding, Phosphorus is a patient who is on fire, and whose catabolic or destructive processes are extremely active. On the mental plane, the personality is destroyed. As in Sulphur, Phosphorus has a large appetite, with sluggishness and weakness in the abdomen, especially at 11 a.m. and a sensation of a prolapsed abdomen. Phosphorus patients must eat frequently to avoid feeling faint; they are hungry after eating and hungry at night, which causes them to get up; they may even feel hungry during a headache; they are averse to sweets, but crave alcohol and salt to excess.

He suffers from constant muscular tension with stiffness on beginning to move and tearing, drawing pains – a paralytic-type syndrome that causes limping and total loss of muscle strength.

Other important symptoms are:

A cough that rises from the stomach after eating, due to a tickling sensation in the pit of the stomach; coughing when a stranger enters the room; coughing when smelling strong odours; and coughing with suffocating retrosternal pains and contraction of the larynx, as if something had broken loose inside.

Hoarseness worse by talking, with constriction and spasm of the larynx.

Constant irritation of the larynx, worse by talking; loss of the voice and hoarseness after talking for a long time or when the weather changes.

Runny nose, panting and laboured breathing, emphysema, asthma after coughing. Headaches with a splitting sensation when coughing.

Sensation of cold in the brain.

Congestion of the head which seems to start in the spinal column.

Congestive head and visual symptoms; letters appear red or patient always sees green. Sees a halo surrounding lights and often colours appear to be black.

Stools are long and hard, like a dog's stools, and are expelled with great difficulty. Profuse, involuntary, painless, bloody diarrhoea, with membranes and blood-like particles and the sensation of the anus remaining open as if there had been no contraction of the sphincter. (One 17-month-old baby boy, in a comatose state, oozed faecal matter out of the anus as if it were an inert orifice; Phosphorus 30c saved him.)

One of this remedy's peculiar modalities is an aggravation of symptoms during thunderstorms. Not only do thunderstorms increase the fear, they also produce muscular pains.

Dusk aggravates the symptoms and, except for the head and stomach, they are generally worse in cold weather and before sleeping, although they will awake from a nap feeling better. Sleeping on the left side does not agree with them. They dislike the contact of clothing on the skin, and are especially sensitive to the pressure of bedclothes. (Phosphorus children will throw their bedclothes off at night.) Hot food and hot drinks, wind, light, music, noise, playing the piano and staying in the dark will all aggravate the symptoms. However, their congestive headaches are better in the open air.

Clinical experience has confirmed that Phosphorus produces a fatty degeneration of the liver and pancreas and a fatty and amyloid degeneration of the kidney. It attacks the hips, knees and left submaxillary and produces caries, exostosis of the spinal column and diabetes.

There are fluctuating states of hyperactivity, vehemence, irascibility, emotional excitement and mental stimulation, followed by a marked paralytic decline. Phosphorus is like a fire which bursts suddenly into flame only to die out shortly after.

A full knowledge of the patient's history will necessarily include his reactions to life's challenges and the nature of his frustrations and family relationships, thus revealing his prevailing constitutional tendency and the way in which he has responded psychologically and physiologically to vital and environmental stimuli.

The current symptom picture cannot be the entire case. The present moment is the epilogue of a long process which can be revealed only by the patient's whole life history. The changes, frustrations and conditions in the patient's life all have an influence on the constitution.

Thus there is a dynamic relationship between the subject and the environment: the organism has its inherent weaknesses and imbalances; the environment moulds the personality and determines the morbid physiopathological processes accordingly.

Symptoms are the symbolic expression of an unconscious vital force which finds its fullest expression of totality in a patient's mental symptoms. These provide an understanding of the way in which each person will react to the same situations. For example, when faced with identical frustrations, Silica will respond with timidity, cowardice and feeling of inferiority; Natrum Muriaticum with resentment, rejection and isolation; Phosphorus with fear and anxiety.

Constitutional

Nerve tissue – Bones – Burning.
Accelerated metabolism, fanning the fire of life.
Right side.

Mental Symptoms

Impulsive; impulse to kill: Iodum, Hepar Sulphuris, Platinum.
Oversensitive, emotional, intuitive, reacts quickly then sinks into apathy.
Indifferent to everything, including family and friends. As in Sepia, indifference towards own children.
Thin, weak.
Acute senses: Arsenicum, Coffea, Belladonna, Nux Vomica, Opium, Phosphorus.
Apathetic; does not pay attention to anything. Answers unwillingly or talks very fast – suddenly breaks off, feels vexed and reacts with great irascibility and vehemence; is capable of killing.
Sympathetic: identifies with others' misfortune, unselfish, feels pity for broken toys. Seeks sympathy, companionship, affection, pampering, understanding, support. Kisses everybody. Dependent personality. Wants company and consolation.
Chaotic.
Restlessness: cannot stay still.
Chronic effects of fright, sadness, grief, nostalgia.
The world seems an unbearable place to be.
Depression of the sensorium, unintelligible chatter, stuporous state, unconscious; when awakened, recovers full consciousness.
Whimsical, sensitive. Refined, presumptuous; children who like to be

well dressed and well groomed. Extremely sensitive, both physically and emotionally.

Fear: of solitude, thunderstorms, death, disease, calamities, burglars, ghosts, darkness. Anxiety at dusk.

Tendency to be emotional.

Bad humour, restlessness and faint-heartedness at dusk.

Anxiety: head and hands feel hot, heart feels closed and oppressed. Anxious about his illness and the future. Imagines faces that peep out of corners or obscene visions that accuse him.

Lack of modesty: wants to undress and walk about naked.

Thinks she is a high-ranking lady of important affairs.

Extreme restlessness, especially during thunderstorms.

Spasmodic fits of weeping and laughter (hysteria).

State of clairvoyance, extasis (mesmerism). Wants to be magnetised.

Likes being rubbed, stroked, petted, holding hands.

Physical Symptoms

Heat and burning sensation in many areas of the body: mouth, stomach, intestines, anus, back, climbing up the back, palm of the hand.

Tall, thin; narrow thorax; consumptive; straight hair; emaciated; dark-haired (Guernsey) or red-haired or blonde (Nash).

Chronic diarrhoea; tendency to diarrhoea; diarrhoea in children with paretic anus.

Severe pneumonia with gangrene.

Craves cold food and drinks; vomits cold water when warmed in the stomach.

Sensitive to light. Nosebleeds.

Sensation of weakness, emptiness in the abdomen, emptiness in the stomach, feels faint from hunger.

Bulimia. Hungry at night.

Night-time cough due to constant tickling in the throat.

Anxiety in the precordial region, feels hungry; better when eating.

Burning heat between the shoulderblades.

Lies on right side, cannot lie on left side, feels palpitations.

Bleeds easily, small wounds bleed copiously; this remedy affects blood and liver similarly.

As in Crotalus Horridus, deficient coagulation; blood is quick to ooze out.

Necrosis of the mandible.

Suffocating sensation.

Lax muscular system.

Extreme tiredness.

Better after a short sleep, as in Sepia, and as opposed to Lachesis.

General restlessness. Zincum has restless feet.

Phosphorus is slow, phlegmatic, calm, stupid. Slowness: Conium Maculatum, Helleborus Niger, Phosphorus, Calcarea Carbonica, Carbo Vegetabilis, Graphites, Opium, Pulsatilla, Sepia.

Craves salt (due to an accelerated metabolism).

Natrum Muriaticum: craves salt, aversion to greasy foods.

Nitricum Acidum: craves salt and greasy foods.

Argentum Nitricum: craves sweets and sugar.

Consumption: hectic fever. Tuberculosis.

Kent: sickly at birth, rapid growth, remains thin during growth. Fragile, anaemic patients who lose weight easily.

Violent palpitations; sanguine; violent and irascible; tendency to bleed easily; petechias, bruises.

Chest and leg symptoms better by heat; stomach and head symptoms better by cold. Better by cold foods.

Coughs when going from warm to cold surroundings, as opposed to Bryonia, who coughs when changing from cold to warm surroundings. Worse from dusk to midnight.

Very excited sexually (satyriasis or nymphomania), but with diminished sexual potency; sexual conflicts.

Children

Fine, translucent skin; blue eyes that sparkle and shine; blondes and redheads. Asthenic. Impressionable, excitable, reacts with speed and enthusiasm. Quick, alert mind. Quick, sharp, keen perception of people's attitudes. New ideas or emotions are exciting but are instantly extinguished; he then sinks into apathy and indifference.

Indifference interrupted by outbursts of excitement and enthusiasm, as if they were sudden blazes.

Shyness, apathetic, tired of life.

Sensitive to electrical and atmospheric changes, thunderstorms may bring on diarrhoea and/or palpitations.

Impressionable, reacts vivaciously and with ire, but calms down and does not hold grudges, as Natrum Muriaticum does.

Fights with other children, but cannot be alone (Natrum Muriaticum).

Excessive mental activity; outbursts of excitement and anger followed by prostration.

Anxious, fears everything, calms down when held by the hand. Comforted by the presence of others.

Alone. Anxiety worse when alone: Arsenicum, Phosphorus.

Apprehension in the stomach: Mezereum, Aurum, Digitalis, Kali Carbonicum, Lycopodium, Phosphorus. Fear which appears to come from the pit of the stomach.

Nervous system: spasms, fibrillar twitchings. Pains like flashes of lightning (locomotor ataxia).

Heat that rises up the spinal column to the neck and vertex (in Picricum Acidum, it goes down the spinal column).

Cirrhosis, jaundice (Crotalus Horridus).

Asthma, spasmodic cough with blood, especially in pneumonias.

Fear of being alone because he may die: Argentum Nitricum, Arsenicum, Kali Carbonicum, Phosphorus.

Stammering from fear.

Similar to Causticum's paresis; antidoted by Causticum.

Similar to Iodum's tuberculosis. (Iodum is hot and better by open air, is not nervous and does not bleed easily as in Phosphorus. Phosphorus takes cold easily and shivers when chilled.)

Complementary remedies: Calcarea Carbonica, Thuja, Fluoricum Acidum, Sanguinaria, Pulsatilla.

Easygoing character, impulsive, very excitable, easily roused; prone to fits.

Ecstasy: Aconitum, Phosphorus, Agaricus Muscarius, Coffea, Lachesis, Opium.

Walking in the moonlight: Romantic. Antimonium Crudum.

Vertigo brought on by smelling flowers: Nux Vomica, Phosphorus, Hyoscyamus.

Extroverted, spontaneous. Natrum Muriaticum is introverted.

Likes people, fears solitude. Imaginative, makes mountains out of molehills.

Hypocrisy: Phosphorus.

Hot flushes; as if warm water were poured over one, an idea occurs vividly.

Anxiety from excitement; anxiety before coitus.

Girls who isolate themselves and are afraid of leaving the house because they fear 'getting lost' (a taboo concerning sexual arousal).

Fear of insanity, fear of death.

Young patients who fear snakes (homosexual fear due to erotic stimulation).

Indifference to relations: Helleborus, Sepia, Phosphorus. (Phosphorus fluctuates between being sympathetic and indifferent to relations). Indifference to her children.

Chapter 29

Psorinum
(1950)

Psorinum is often indicated in those chronic cases where the well-chosen remedy does not act or when improvement is temporary.

It can act as an intercurrent remedy to clarify the underlying symptom picture. Sulphur is the indicated remedy in acute cases that do not resolve as long as no other remedy is indicated. When Sulphur does not act, Psorinum may be indicated.

Like all nosodes and other remedies of the materia medica, Psorinum must be diagnosed according to the individualising symptoms.

Psorinum is extremely sensitive to cold and weather changes, and catches cold or feels chilly if the head is exposed.

As in Phosphorus, Psorinum feels much restlessness and malaise before thunderstorms. All symptoms are worse in winter – especially the skin eruptions, which disappear in summer.

One peculiar symptom is a fetid body odour, even after bathing. All discharges such as stools, leucorrhoea, menstrual blood and perspiration smell like rotten flesh.

Psorinum is useful when there has been suppression of skin eruptions, diarrhoea or emotions.

He feels unusually well before a crisis, whether it be an asthma attack, diarrhoea, a rash or any acute disease.

On a mental level he is nervous, easily startled and restless, full of fear, anxiety, forebodings, and pessimism.

Psorinum despairs of recovery, of salvation and of success. He makes life intolerable for others with his continual acrimonious and bitter complaints.

Other peculiar symptoms are:

Headaches with hunger which, like Anacardium and Kali Phosphoricum, improve while eating. Psorinum's headaches are generally brought on by suppressed eruptions or menses. As in Melilotus, these headaches improve with a nosebleed and, as in Lac Defloratum and

Kali Bichromicum, are often preceded by dullness and seeing sparks, flies or rings.

Like Lycopodium, the hair lacks lustre, is dry, brittle and tangles easily.

As in Graphites and Mezereum, the scalp is dry, has dandruff and offensive, suppurating, sticky eruptions.

Very sensitive to light, eyelids are very inflamed.

Humid eruptions with fetid, crusty discharges inside and behind the ears. Extremely fetid, chronic thin watery discharge from the ears after a bout of measles or scarlet fever.

Psorinum patients get up at midnight or early dawn to eat, and always have a snack on top of the night-table to eat as soon as they wake up in the morning. Phosphorus, Lycopodium, China and, to a lesser degree, Ignatia share this symptom.

As in Arnica, Antimonium Tartaricum, Agaricus, Sepia and Sulphur, Psorinum has offensive eructations which smell like rotten eggs.

Enlarged tonsils, with repeated inflammation with intense burning pains, much salivation and copious catarrh of the throat which causes constant clearing of the throat. As in Kali Muriaticum, Psorinum will often expel putrid-smelling and putrid-tasting particles from the tonsils.

As in Sulphur, Aloe, Kali Bichromicum, Lilium Tigrinum, Phosphorus, Podophyllum, Rumex, Silica, Tuberculinum and Zincum, Psorinum has a sudden urging for diarrhoea, forcing the patient to jump out of bed in the morning. Stools are watery, dark-yellowish, offensive, smelling like rotten flesh and tend to be passed involuntarily, often after acute diseases, during teething or when the weather changes before a thunderstorm. Psorinum patients tend to feel worse between 1 and 4 a.m.

Diarrhoea alternates with constipation, with inactivity of the rectum like Silica. The bladder is paretic and there is nocturnal incontinence or enuresis.

As an antisycotic remedy, Psorinum is often the intercurrent in stubborn cases of chronic gonorrhoea that do not respond to the constitutional remedy.

In women, Psorinum is useful when there is profuse, offensive leucorrhoea, with general weakness and pains in the sacrolumbar region. It is very useful in pregnancy, especially when there is involuntary vomiting and violent movements of the foetus. When administered in this way, the baby's psoric diathesis is corrected in time.

Unlike Arsenicum, the asthma and bronchitis of Psorinum are worse in the open air and when sitting down; better by lying down with the arms outspread. There is despair of recovery, with the sensation that he is dying.

Coughing returns every winter along with the rest of the symptoms. Allergic symptoms of the skin or mucous membranes reappear at the same time of year, and the patient can tell the physician the precise time at which his symptoms will come back.

If the patient is treated throughout the winter it is possible to eradicate the underlying diathesis in future years.

As in Phosphorus and Tuberculinum, the cough is particularly violent in the morning on waking and at night before retiring. Yellowish-green, salty sputum is often present. The cough follows the suppression of a skin eruption or eczema.

Like Sulphur, there is a tendency towards eczematous eruptions which may look like impetigo, as in Hepar Sulphuris. The skin is dry with no perspiration and looks dirty, as if the patient never washed. The face will often have a thin coat of seborrhoea, which makes the skin look greasy. These are sad, depressed, despairing, discouraged patients who are sensitive to cold, dirty, unkempt, with bad breath and disagreeable body odour, and dry or scaly skin eruptions that force them constantly to scratch.

Chapter 30

Sepia
(1955)

Sepia's main feature is emotional indifference. Sepia patients are capable of feeling no affection for their family, spouse, children or close friends. They are indifferent and apathetic, not only towards their loved ones but also about their job and home. Sepia does not care what happens, does not want to take charge of anything and feels that life has lost its meaning.

The patient shows a marked decrease in mental ability. The face is inexpressive and torpid, and thinking is too much of an effort. Speech is slow as he gropes for the right words.

Two features that stand out in this remedy are sadness and irritability.

Sepia women feel miserable and suffer from fits of bitter weeping. They are unhappy about everything and feel utterly wretched about their illness. They are listless, full of fears and easily frightened by noise and other sensory impressions. Life holds no attraction for them whatsoever – they have lost interest in everything.

Irritability alternates with depression and indifference. There are outbursts of passionate irritability at the slightest provocation, a petty offence, a supposed vexation or a trivial contradiction. Sepia will explode in violent outbursts of rage with furious gesticulations. Hysteria alternates with the most contrary moods.

The mental symptom picture of Sepia can be illustrated more vividly with a real life case. A 30-year-old mother had an obsessive fear of harming her two children, aged two and four years. She had a bad relationship with her husband and would attack him at the slightest provocation. She was exasperated by her husband's mental stability, as she was so unbalanced herself. She needed her husband but was not sexually attracted to him. She would reproach him for not pampering her and then would feel bad for being so demanding, as she knew that she asked for a lot but gave nothing in return.

She felt guilty for her selfishness and her detachment. She had no faith in life. Her husband was an angel, she said, but she did not love him. She would weep on seeing her children because she feared she might harm them and would desperately spoil them to compensate for her lack of love.

She said that it was as if all her love had turned into hate, and she hated herself for harbouring these bad feelings. She felt guilty for being so unfair and mean, so incapable of real emotion or of reciprocating all the love and affection everybody gave her. It was terrible, she said, always to be owing ... and then she would burst into tears.

She was emotionally and sexually frigid. She felt torn between her self-centredness and her guilty conscience that reproached her for not fulfilling her duty towards others. In so doing, her conscience was pointing out to her how she was transgressing Hering's law – that is, evolving from centre to periphery, from individual to world, from I to we, from selfishness to altruism.

In the physiological and spiritual evolution of the human being, the law of cure is fulfilled when, as Jung said, self-serving interests become transcended into love for others and for divinity. When the vital impulse does not follow this path, illness, both mental and physical, will be the result.

This mental symptom picture is associated with congestion and eventual prolapse of the abdominal and pelvic organs; she complained of heaviness in the lower abdomen, with a bearing-down sensation in the pelvic region, a sensation of prolapse with drawing pains in the sacro-lumbar region, as if the suspensory ligaments of the womb were being pulled.

This genital syndrome is caused by congestion of the abdominal organs, especially in the branches of the portal vein, followed by a prolapsed uterus, a sensation of hunger in the stomach, a sensation of having a ball in the rectum, polyuria with incontinence, hot flushes, pain and heaviness in the lower back, pains in the joints, and sluggishness of the lower limbs from venous stasis and aggravated by standing.

The most important aspect of this pelvic symptom picture is its influence on the genital functions and on sexual frigidity, which is both characteristic of pelvic weakness and the physical reflection of emotional indifference. Sepia becomes withdrawn both emotionally and sexually. In this way, mental symptoms find their correlation on a physical level.

The link which unites the contrasting manifestations of Sepia's lack of vital strength is the autonomic nervous system, which transmits impulses from the cellular level to the highest levels of mental function.

The autonomic nervous system – more accurately termed the life of the unconscious – coordinates and harmonises every part of the body, from the cell to the neurons of the cerebral cortex, and facilitates individual behaviour.

The biological requirements of the cell are transmitted to the autonomic nervous system which, through synapsis with the nerve fibres from the whole organism, is correlated to the organic whole; from the small centres of the sympathetic ganglia through higher levels of integration to the centres of the mesencephalon, wherein every organic function is represented. The centres of the diencephalon, the hypothalamus and the pituitary gland, which controls the endocrine system, exchange messages with the cerebral cortex so that the entire nervous system forms a continuous whole working in harmony.

The higher nerve centres control and energise the lower ones so that chemical processes can take place at the cellular level. The instinctive aspects of behaviour are controlled by the mesencephalic level, the cortical centres or higher levels of intelligence, consciousness and spirit.

This whole complex system coordinates and energises the psychic life of the individual, allowing the most basic and the most complex processes to take place, from the unconscious phenomena of organic life to the highest form of conscious spiritual activity.

It is necessary, however, to make a distinction between the terms psyche or psychic and mind or mental. The psyche includes both the conscious and unconscious mind, whereas the mind refers only to the conscious mind.

In homoeopathy we use the term 'mental symptoms' incorrectly, because they really refer to unconscious phenomena which become conscious when activated in the patient's personality. It would be more accurate to speak of psychic rather than mental symptoms, because they involve the expression of the organism's whole physiology, have their own physical structure and are subject to the same physiological laws.

The mental refers to the ego, that is, consciousness of the self and the world; the psychic is that which mediates between the inner world of needs, instincts, emotions and feelings, and the outer world of the patient's social environment.

Homoeopathic medicine takes into account both the psychic symptoms – moods, feelings and emotional drives – and the mental symptoms that arise from the personality conflicts between primitive instinct and life experience.

However, the most revealing thing about the patient is the way he manages to adapt to reality and resolve the conflict between his inner and outer worlds. Why is this so? Because the individual's ego is un-balanced and therefore diseased; that is, because its capacity for syn-thesis has been deranged and therefore rendered incapable of adapting to life.

By studying both the character and behaviour of the ego, through a comprehensive inquiry into the patient's life history, the physician will be able to discern the psychic symptoms which express the emotional state that makes up the patient's innermost self, his unconscious will or morbid dynamic tendency.

A patient will mask, modify or even hide symptoms of the psyche, because of the anxiety generated by the conflict between instinctual impulses and the need to be socially acceptable. Primitive instincts are suppressed and relegated to the psychic unconscious and organs of the body, thus causing organ symptoms or neurosis which, with or without pathology, contain the patient's anxiety.

When psychic energies are too intense, or when the possibility of release is thwarted by the external world or by internal censorship, a transformation takes place in the different layers of the personality or psychic-organic strata.

We have seen that behind Lycopodium's façade of haughtiness, pride, misanthropy, disdainful indifference and domineering attitude, lies a deep, hidden lack of self-confidence, a trepidation and timidity which fills him with anxiety due to the conflict between what he wants to be but cannot, between his desire for self-affirmation and what is permitted by society. In contrast, Sepia's anxiety is caused by the conflict between the active, masculine-oriented desire for success and self-affirmation, and the emotional coldness or inability to give affec-tion, which is an essentially passive, feminine trait. This is why Sepia is generally a female remedy. While Lycopodium's conflict is one of active self-affirmation, Sepia's conflict is one of passive, emotional and sexual giving.

In women, sexual activity is a psychological and physical experience which activates the whole being. Essentially sexuality has elements of both selfishness and altruism, narcissistic self-love and love for others.

Throughout the sexual development of both men and women, there is a constant wavering between the active impulses of aggression or domination and those of receptivity, dependency or passivity. Thus, the personality is capable of both aggressiveness and subordination. Although this conflict is present in every human being, it is an out-standing feature in Lycopodium men and in Sepia women, bearing in mind, of course, that each have both masculine and feminine components to some degree.

In Sepia, emotional and sexual frigidity manifests as aggressiveness, anxiety and self-reproach. The root of Sepia's coldness stems from a profound weakness of the psyche.

The syndrome of passive pelvic congestion with prolapsed genital organs does not necessarily indicate Sepia. Murex Purpurea, Lilium Tigrinum and Platinum also have prolapse and plethora of the portal vein; however, nymphomania or sexual excitement are present in these remedies.

Sepia's sexual frigidity is intimately connected to emotional frigidity and intense anger.

Fundamentally, sexual frigidity is a biological phenomenon that can best be understood through a complete knowledge of the patient's life history. Frigidity has different causes which the physician must be familiar with:

1) Improper sexual education, or unconscious moral prejudices which forbid sexuality and view it as sinful and something which should be punished.

2) An unconscious resentment against men, in order to avenge the mother for the suffering inflicted upon her by a brutal father.

3) A high masculine component and a lifelong feeling of inferiority to men.

4) Childish emotional fixation on the father; immaturity, self-centredness, narcissism, exclusive self-love, thus rendering the patient incapable of experiencing the feelings of a mature woman.

Mental Symptoms

Very easily offended and inclined to anger.
Fits of weeping and involuntary laughter.
Afraid to be alone.
Very sensitive to the slightest noise.
Anxiety, hot flushes in the face; fear concerning real or imaginary ills.
Annoyed by any kind of work.
Contrary, quarrelsome, complains of everything.
Passionate, irritable.
Bad memory. When speaking, forgets main points.
Muddled and obtuse thinking.
Indolent, distracted, inattentive.
Industrious.

Life seems meaningless.
Desire to weep all the time, without knowing why.
Very sad, apathetic. Worse when walking in open air and at dusk.
Unsatisfied with everything. Sad concerning health and household tasks. Sad, sombre. Feels unfortunate without a cause.
Tendency to suicide, feels desperate about his miserable existence.
So enraged that he fears apoplexy. Everything turns black before the eyes.
Passionate outbursts with trembling, worse in the hands, at the slightest trifle.
Ire with much excitement, does not know what to do.
Aversion to company.
Lacks ambition. Does not want to work, or have fun, or make the slightest mental effort.
Becomes bad-tempered when thinking of past disagreeable events.
Aversion to homoeopathy (Gallavardin).

The Sepia mentality may be found even in women who have deceptively soft, sweet characters, but the most frequent sign is a guilty resentment of her children, with feelings of revulsion for her poor, well-meaning husband and the desire to be left alone at home.

Enjoys watching thunderstorms, which ameliorate sadness.

Thunderstorms, rainy or cloudy days ameliorate; enlivened by atmospheric electricity, general debility and muscle weakness is ameliorated.

Abdomen

Pressure and heaviness in the abdomen with a sensation of expansion as if it were about to burst. Excessive abdominal distension with movements and rumbling; flatulence; trapped wind.
Colic with urges to defecate, stabbing pains.
Pinching pains in the groin.

Female Genitalia

Protrusion of the uterus, sharp, stabbing pains which shoot upwards; colic before menstruation.

Male Genitalia

Profuse perspiration in the genitals, especially the scrotum. Warts on the margin of the prepuce. Pseudogonorrhoea. Ulcers of the glans and prepuce. Cutting pains in the testicles. Swollen testicles, weakness of the genital organs.

Increased sexual desire with constant erections, especially at night. Frequent ejaculations.

Discharge of prostatic fluid before urinating and while defecating.

Mental, emotional and physical fatigue after coitus and ejaculation.

Worse after coitus.

In men, sensation of distension or languor of the stomach after defecating (observed). Pains associated with inguinal hernia and in the lumbar region which improve by lifting the abdomen with the hand (observed, Dr Leo).

In women, dyspareunia, painful or irritating coitus, sometimes with vaginismus.

Sexual frigidity, disaffected. Seeks some occupation 'to have a reason to live'. Ameliorated by occupation because she feels no joy or sexual desire.

Chapter 31

Silica
(1956)

Silica is a mineral which gives hardness, consistency and solidity to nature. Sand, quartz, stone, flint and gravel all give hardness to steel, glass, diamonds and everything in nature that requires solidity and resistance. It gives firmness to the fibre in plant stalks and animal tissue; it is the main constituent of the connective tissue of the skin, hair, nails and bones. In the human being, silica provides firmness and consistency to the physical structure and integrity, fortitude and energy to the spirit. Hence, the symptom picture features weakness and a lack of backbone – like a building constructed without sand.

The average amount of silica in the body is only sixty or seventy grams; hence its role is as a catalyst of biological processes rather than a chemical substance. Any disturbances in metabolic and assimilation processes are due to constitutional dynamic factors. Silica is one of many inorganic elements in the body that does not produce individualising symptoms; it is not through an inquiry into the chemical mechanism of metabolic disturbance that we will be led to diagnose Silica, nor for that matter any other remedy in the materia medica. The diagnosis must be based on the characteristic totality of symptoms which represent the patient's disease and forms the true image of the remedy. A slow-acting remedy, Silica develops its symptoms over a long period of time and is indicated in deep-seated hereditary conditions.

Generally speaking, Silica is a lymphatic, tubercular-sycotic remedy with irritability of the nervous system as in Nux Vomica. Silica patients are sad, fearful and anxious, lacking spirit and energy. They are emaciated with poor assimilation, weakness, sensitivity to the cold and to external stimuli. The nails are brittle and break easily. The heads and feet perspire profusely and there is a tendency to suppuration.

Silica children are thin with large heads and abdomens. They tend to be short, thin and slow to walk. The fontanelles are slow to close. The skin is cold and yellowish, the ganglia are enlarged and indurated and the bones tend to curve. Wounds are slow to heal, suppurate easily and have a tendency to produce fistulae. Foot-sweat, and head-sweat which soaks the pillow, are common.

Silica suffers from an irritable weakness with hyperaesthesia, hypersensitivity and intense anxiety. Shyness, fearfulness, depression, docility, compliance and lethargy alternate with irritability, rage, shouting, screaming and hostility, or with stubbornness, obstinacy and inflexibility.

Physical and mental weakness with hypersensitivity and irritability.

Mental Symptoms

Lacks stamina, vitality, fibre, nerve, vigour, backbone; weak character, cowardly, fearful, embarrassed, weeps every evening.

Pale, yellowish, fearful, nervous, easily discouraged, apathetic, very sensitive to noise and touch; guilt, sadness. Irritable with fits of rage. Stubborn, discontented.

Sad, melancholy, taciturn children. Children who feel they are going to die.

Lacking in spirit. Weak character, like Lycopodium and Causticum. Timid, docile, accommodating, disturbed, anxious and agitated, with a fit of anxiety, fear, terror, dread waking.

Adult, intellectual, intelligent, professional people; patients who come to the doctor's office exhausted from prolonged mental exertion and the stress of public appearances, with much nervousness before the event and fear of failing, as in students before an exam. When faced with appearing in public or taking an exam, Silica patients are afraid of being unable to coordinate their ideas or find the right words to express themselves, as in Gelsemium. However, they are capable of conquering their fear and performing with brilliance and precision because their inability is only imagined; whereas in Lycopodium the fears are based on real inadequacy.

Mentally exhausted students who have completed their studies after extraordinary efforts and who feel incapable of practising their profession, for fear of failure. Similarly, employees of a company who feel incapable of carrying on with their work, as if their brains had been stretched to the limit.

Weeps as soon as someone says something to him; weeps when spoken to with affection. Stubborn, obstinate, discontented. Homesickness.

Extreme irritability. Irritable, bad-tempered and timid. Easily angered. Fits of rage, but not as violent as in Calcarea Carbonica. Must restrain his violent impulses.

Very sensitive to noise. Startled by noise, becomes anxious and screams, cannot bear to be spoken to in a loud voice. Starting. Painful sensitivity in the ears caused by loud noises.

Extremely scrupulous. Conscientious, meticulous, careful.

Conscientious about trifles with irresolution.

Anxiety of conscience. Obsessive, as if guilty of a bad deed, a terrible offence, the biggest crime.

Restless, impatient, does not know what to do.

Tired of life, apathetic, indifferent; nervous debility with abnormal sensitivity.

Sensitive to touch. Lacks serenity.

Has the sensation of being in two different places at once.

Weeps on telling her symptoms: Silica, Pulsatilla, Sepia, Kali Carbonicum, Medorrhinum.

Mentally active, intelligent, but no inclination for mental work.

Does not want to make any mental effort. Becomes tired on reading, writing, thinking or meditating.

Makes the same mistakes over and over again when studying. Makes mistakes when speaking.

Weak memory, distracted. Finds it difficult to focus attention; even short conversations are exhausting.

Constant fainting. Epilepsy; sleepwalking at new and full moons.

Selfishness.

Avarice: Arsenicum, Lycopodium, Pulsatilla, Sepia, Silica.

Hypocrite, sly, cunning.

Fearful.

Obstinate, stubborn.

Very susceptible.

Priggish: Platinum, Pulsatilla, Silica.

Hasty, always in a hurry.

Impatient.

Servile and obsequious.

Minutely precise.

Unfit for singing, painting and commerce.

Dunham: When forced to carry out a task, Silica will work far beyond his limits until utterly fatigued.

Fixed ideas about pins. Afraid of pins, but looks for them and gathers them together carefully.

Anticipation: Anxiety as if something were expected of him. Nervous when having to go somewhere and fulfil a commitment. Anxiety from anticipation. Feelings of inferiority.

Anxiety before examinations: Aconitum, Aethusa Cynapium, Anacardium Orientale, Argentum Nitricum, Borax, Bryonia, Camphora, Causticum, Carcinosin, Cicuta Virosa, Coffea, Fluoricum Acidum, Gelsemium, Graphites, Hyoscyamus, Ignatia, Lac Caninum, Lycopodium, Medorrhinum, Mercurius, Natrum Carbonicum, Natrum Muriaticum, Nux Vomica, Petroleum, Phosphoricum Acidum, Phosphorus, Plumbum, Pulsatilla, Silica, Staphysagria, Stillingia, Strontium, Thuja, Veratrum.

Anxiety anticipating an engagement: Argentum Nitricum, Gelsemium, Medorrhinum.

Anxiety when anything is expected of him: Arsenicum Album.

Timidity appearing in public: Carbo Vegetabilis, Gelsemium, Plumbum, Silica.

Fear of failure: Psorinum, Silica.

State of apathy, mental debility and fear of failure and of appearing in public after a great mental effort.

Anxiety of conscience (as if guilty of a crime). Hides sexual passions during puberty and believes himself to be guilty of obscene or evil acts. (Sycosis: Medorrhinum, Thuja.) Alumina, Arsenicum, Aurum, Chelidonium, Digitalis, Psorinum.

Physical Symptoms

Silica acts on the connective tissue, ganglia, mucous membranes, skin, hair and nail. Illness brought on by suppressed discharges or perspiration, cracks, fissures and fistulae.

All secretions are fetid, watery and acrid, with a smell of dead flesh.

Scrofulous appearance with enlarged ganglia in the neck, armpits and groin that itch rather than hurt.

Malnourished, atrophied, hypersensitive, dry skin with easy bruising; wounds take a long time to heal.

Marasmus. Poor nutrition. Thin children with good appetites: Silica, Abrotanum, Natrum Muriaticum, Sulphur, Calcarea, Iodum.

Children who are sluggish, psoric, scrofulous. Old-looking, sunken face. Thin legs. Stunted growth and development.

Thin, syphilitic-psoric children who perspire on the head during sleep and have weak ankles. Newborn babies with big heads and open fontanelles, as in Calcarea Carbonica.

Selfish, hypersensitive, thin children who are malnourished because of faulty assimilation, not a lack of food, which may lead to an emaciated state as in Lycopodium, Natrum Muriaticum and Phosphorus.

Cold sensation, with much sensitivity to cold. Lack of vital heat.
This is a left-sided remedy.

Immunisation: For the side effects of smallpox vaccine, convulsions.
Thuja, with diarrhoea and eruptions.
Malandrinum, with chronic skin symptoms.

Head

Damp, scaly, itchy, eczematous eruptions, with offensive discharges.
Eczema with fetid discharges in children. Copious perspiration of the
head during sleep and pains. Open fontanelles. Headaches that begin in
the nape of the neck and settle in the supraorbital region on the right
side, better by heat. Supraorbital pains that improve with pressure and
local heat. Pain and sensation of cold, better by wrapping the head and
conserving warmth. Sensation of heaviness in the neck.

Headaches once a week with vertigo, nausea and vomiting.

Vertigo that begins in the spinal column and rises through the occiput
to the forehead, with a sensation of falling forward.

Hot flushes of the head with a red, burning face. Bloody, congested
nose. The head feels as if it could not be held.

Headache that starts in the spinal column, shoots up through the nape
of the neck and occiput and settles in the right vertex or right eye. (On
the left eye: Spigelia.)

Headache that feels as if the head were about to explode, better by
binding the head tightly.

The head is sensitive to touch, feels hot, congested.

Profuse and fetid perspiration of the whole head and face. (Calcarea
Carbonica perspires only on the scalp.)

Eyes

Blepharitis with oedema, reddening and suppuration of the rim of the
eyelids. Chalazion and styes. Inflamed, suppurating tear ducts, fistulae
of tear ducts. Intense photophobia is usually present. Iriditis and
coroiditis with pus in the anterior chamber of the eye. Scrofulous
ophthalmia with a tendency to develop perforation of the cornea.

Swollen tear duct, obstructed tear ducts, the eye waters constantly.

Ears

Hypersensitivity to noise. Catarrhal otitis of the eardrum and eustachian
tube, with deafness, and a sudden onset of catarrh from the eardrum

215

to the eustachian tube; roaring sensation. Chronic otorrhoea, with thick, crusty, fetid pus, with caries of the mastoid cells and small bones.

Eczema behind the ear. Spasmodic cough when picking the ear.

Face

A pale, waxy, transparent complexion, with acne around the nostrils and chin.

The face sweats with the slightest exertion, even though the rest of the body may not perspire.

Perspiration mainly on the head and upper part of the body.

Intense headaches and pains of the eyes, teeth and ears, aggravated by humidity. Heightening of all senses before the pains with chilliness and pallor.

Mouth

Sensation of a hair on the tongue.
Mouth ulcers.

Stomach

Aversion to meat. Indigestion from eating meat.

Craves milk but not cold milk, as opposed to Phosphorus and Tuberculinum. Silica babies may reject their mothers' milk. Milk aggravates. When mother's milk causes diarrhoea: Natrum Carbonicum or Silica, not Aethusa.

Rectum

Constipation with ineffectual urging and inactivity of the rectum. Anus feels constricted.

Bleeding of the anus. Painful haemorrhoids; anal fissures and fistulae.

As in Sanicula and Thuja, stools in children recede after being partially expelled.

Anal fistulae (Fluoricum Acidum, Hepar Sulphuris, Mercurius).

Diarrhoea from anticipation: Argentum Nitricum, Gelsemium, Phosphoricum Acidum.

Diarrhoea from excitement as before theatre: Argentum Nitricum.

Diarrhoea from excitement: Argentum Nitricum, Gelsemium, Phosphoricum Acidum, Thuja.

Diarrhoea from exciting news: Gelsemium.

Sleep

Insomnia with congestion and heat in the head and palpitations. Restlessness with anxiety, horrible dreams and nightmares. Perspires upon falling asleep. Sleepwalking; gets up, walks about and goes back to sleep.

Sleeps in the foetal position. The position the patient sleeps in is very important. The following remedies sleep in the knee-chest position with the head buried in the pillow: Carcinosin, Medorrhinum, Calcarea Phosphorica, Natrum Muriaticum, Phosphorus, Sepia.

Extremities

Offensive odour of the feet without perspiration: Graphites, Sepia, Silica.

Fetid foot-sweat, with itchy excoriation between the toes. Sensitivity of the soles of the feet.

Sensation as if a suppuration or felon were about to appear on the fingertips.

Weakness of the legs.

Slouches when walking, flat-footed, bow-legged.

Hands hot at night, in bed.

Skin

Constitutional: connective tissue and suppuration. Fistulae, boils, fatty cysts, pustules, abscesses, indurated tissues, keloids on scars, fibrous cysts and nodules, ulcers that scar with induration.

Silica promotes keloid suppuration and normal scarring. Keloids that itch when warm.

Small wounds suppurate or heal slowly; coppery, shrivelled skin.

Pustulating acne on the forehead, trunk and sternum.

Ulcers around the nails.

Fever

Sensitive to cold; feels chills and shivers easily, even when exercising.

Sensitive to air currents or when uncovering the head or feet, as in Psorinum. Sleeps covered up to the head, in the foetal position, although may throw the covers off when feeling hot, as in Sulphur.

Profuse perspiration towards dawn. Perspiration of the head. Perspiration has putrid, cadaver-like odour. Perspiration during sleep: Calcarea Carbonica, Calcarea Phosphorica, Chamomilla, Mercurius, Sepia, Silica.

While Calcarea perspires only on the head, Silica perspires on the head, neck and face.

Modalities

Aggravation from cold, being in open air, during winter, from getting chilled on rising in the morning, from cold and damp, after a bath, at full moon and new moon, and during menstrual periods.

Better by dry cold. Lack of vital heat.

Worse by heat, in a warm room. Suffocation in a warm room (acute or chronic fevers).

Desire for and better from open air.

As in Phosphorus, wishes to be magnetised, which ameliorates.

Antidotes: Mercurius, Hepar Sulphuris, Fluoricum Acidum.

Complementary remedies: Pulsatilla, Thuja, Sanicula.

Chapter 32

Syphilinum
(1955)

Syphilinum (Luesinum or Lueticum) is a nosode prepared from the syphilis bacterium.

In syphilitic affections, when a well-prescribed remedy fails to produce a reaction, Syphilinum, applied aetiologically and isopathically, mobilises the organism and triggers the emergence of a symptom picture which may call for any remedy in the materia medica. Apart from this, Syphilinum is a remedy just like any other, with its own symptom picture, and must be prescribed according to the Law of Similars.

Syphilinum, then, belongs to the group of remedies which are indicated in syphilitic cases, although the heavy metals such as gold, lead and mercury also have enormous destructive power because of their high atomic weight – destruction being an essential keynote of syphilis. This raises an important point. The spirochaete is a carrier of syphilis but it is not the only factor in this disease, as syphilis is a dynamic reaction of the whole organism to a dynamic morbific factor.

In syphilis, the specific action is destruction. Gold, lead, arsenic, mercury and iodine are antisyphilitic because their ionic activity generates a destructive action such as that of syphilis. Thus, they can produce a disease with a deeper and more complete symptom picture than the original disease. Let us not forget that the nature of disease is dynamic and also Hahnemann's recognition that disease comes from a disturbance of the vital force – the germ is a by-product of disease.

The real nature of the disease, then, lies in the specific emotional disturbance of the individual. No wonder the statement that the affective is what is most effective in human beings is so relevant to modern clinical practice.

Furthermore, the tertiary symptoms of syphilis, brought about by the suppression of the symptoms by drugs, give limited information on the nature of the disease. Conventional medicine overlooks an enormous amount of unidentified pathological symptoms of the disease which it does not recognise as being characteristically syphilitic. The dynamic symptoms and constitutional symptom pictures of the materia medica go far beyond the scope of the spirochaete and the reactions observed by Wasserman, Kahn and Nelson. These symptoms explain why syphilis is a tubercular manifestation without reference to Koch's bacillus, and why sycosis is more than just *Neisseia gonorrhoeae* and is linked to other vaccine-related toxins.

Syphilinum's main feature is that all symptoms are aggravated at night. Pains, headaches, asthma, rheumatism and other ills are all aggravated at dusk and better at sunrise; on waking, the patient feels terribly exhausted, both mentally and physically. There is an intense fear of nightfall, of becoming insane or paralysed. At dusk the pains intensify, leading to insomnia, restlessness and anxiety while he prays for daylight. The thought of death – syphilitic destruction – taken to its limit, is welcomed as a release from an intolerable night.

Syphilinum patients are irritable, violent and very bad-tempered, angry because they are unable to concentrate on reading, studying or performing calculations. There is significant memory loss of names, places or dates. A curious fact is that although the short-term memory fails, the long-term memory remains intact. This coincides with the period when the patient either contracted syphilis or when the disease became active. There is a notably great clumsiness and incomprehension during the consultation.

The cerebral action of syphilis diminishes the intelligence and memory, and patients become apathetic and indifferent, hopeless of recovery and intolerant of all others' attempts at consolation. They become excited at the slightest contradiction, weep convulsively with rage, and then become distracted, absorbed and obsessive about washing their hands. Syphilis has great irritability, as seen in syphilitic infants who cry furiously without ceasing from the time they are born, and in adults who can't stop washing their hands as a reaction to their unconscious fear and aggression.

There is a deterioration of the intelligence and the ability for positive expression, and the patient's personality is destroyed. Aurum is restrained by an accusing guilty conscience; Mercurius is agitated, anxious and capable of killing, and wishes to run away, to escape from himself. Syphilinum destroys intelligence and the ability to understand, causes mental prostration and softening of the brain.

The destruction of syphilis reaches from the highest level of cerebral function to every organ and tissue of the body.

Dry, wrinkled, marasmic, poorly-nourished children with old-looking, bad-tempered faces; ophthalmia in newborn babies, in contrast to the fat, hydrogenoid, large-headed sycotic patients.

Ulcers, necrosis and abscesses of the mouth, eyes, nose and ears, genitalia and skin.

Recurring abscesses are a salient feature. When a patient has a history of recurring abscesses or suppurations, two remedies to be considered are Syphilinum and Pyrogenium.

Pyrogenium is a syphilitic nosode, made from decayed ox meat. It is similar to Arsenicum, and is an agitated, anxious remedy who believes in its delirious state that its limbs are separate from the body and spread out over the bed, as in Baptisia. Foul, syphilitic breath, very offensive excretions and discharges.

Syphilitic wandering pains that start and disappear slowly.

Head

The syphilitic headache is well known as a line of pain that shoots from one eye to the other, or from one temporal fossa to the other, or from both frontal lobes in a parallel line behind the occiput, a symptom which could well precede an epileptic seizure.

Stabbing pains in the occipital region; full, dull, heavy sensation from the base of the brain to the cerebellum. Pains worse at night; hair falls out.

Carotid ganglia which denotes syphilitic and tubercular adenoma. Dirty, fetid, oozing eczema of the scalp.

Eyes

Acute ophthalmia in newborns. Red eyes which secrete pus, swollen eyelids.

Conjunctivitis in older children, with intense pains, photophobia and watering of the eyes followed by iritis which aggravates the pains between 2 a.m. and 5 a.m.

Patient wakes up with eyelids stuck together and oedema of the upper eyelids.

Phlyctenular conjunctivitis with a chronic recurrence of pustules and inflammation of the cornea in scrofulous children.

Syphilitic inflammation of the eye, conjunctivitis, interstitial keratitis and iritis all worsen after midnight. Burning, watery eyes, intense photophobia and sharp pains.

Paralysis of the orbicular and palpebral muscles, leading to strabismus, drooping of the upper eyelid and paralysis of the upper oblique.

Rheumatic ophthalmia with red conjunctiva, chemosis, sensation of sand in the eyes, eyelids that stick overnight, copious watering, intense photophobia and pains in the head and face, worse from 3–4 a.m.

Papular and vesicular rash of the inner angle of the left eye, nose, cheek and eyebrow with sticky eyelids.

Ears

Suppurating otitis with profuse discharge. Progressive deafness.

Nose

Rhinitis with fetid greenish-yellow discharge. Syphilitic ozaena. Chronic obstruction of the nasal fossae.

Face

Partial paralysis of the right side of the face. Tics and spasmodic contractions of muscles, as in Parkinson's disease.

Mouth

Eczematous eruptions. Small, irregular, triangular, low-cut teeth with caries in the gumline.

Thick, red, fissured tongue. Tongue feels paralysed; difficulty in talking.

Teeth leave marks on sides of tongue.

Foul breath. Profuse, viscous, stringy salivation. Fetid, putrid breath is characteristic of syphilis and tuberculosis.

Putrid taste in the mouth before an epileptic fit.

Ulcers, thrush on the gums, tongue and the inside of the cheeks and lips.

Syphilitic destruction of the soft and hard palate.

All symptoms worse at night.

Throat

Chronic enlargement of the tonsils. Adenoid growths.

Appetite

Total and persistent anorexia in children. Aversion to meat. Tendency towards alcoholism.

Stomach

Hyperchlorhydria with heartburn; burning sensation. Ulcers of the stomach or duodenum.

Buboes of the groin. Stubborn, chronic constipation. Dark, fetid faecal matter. Bilious diarrhoea, worse by the seashore, feeling urges to defecate at 5 a.m. Fissures of the anus and rectum.

Urinary Organs

Polyuria at night and oliguria during the day. Slow, feeble urination; must make an effort to urinate. Burning urine. Urethral itch.

Male Sexual Organs

Chancre of the penis with burning pains. Buboes and infarcted inguinal ganglia. Inflammation and induration of the spermatic cord.

Female Sexual Organs

Thick, profuse, yellow, fetid leucorrhoea which spills out of the sanitary pad and runs down the legs (Alumina). Acrid, mucopurulent discharge which excoriates female children's genitalia, accompanied by inflammatory itch, better during menstruation. Heavy, painful periods which come too soon. Pains in the ovaries. Tendency to miscarriage.

Respiratory System

Hoarseness and almost complete loss of voice before menstruation. Syphilitic lesion of the laryngeal cartilage. Chronic asthma worse in the summer, in damp, hot weather and better during the day. Violent asthma attacks from 1–4 a.m. Dry cough with a rough, raw feeling in the throat at night. Whooping cough with violent vomiting. Greyish-greenish-yellowish purulent expectoration. Chest feels oppressed, as if the sternum were sunken; pains in the chest and respiratory distress.

Heart

Piercing pains from the base to the tip, at night. (In reverse order, from the tip to the base, Medorrhinum, and from the base to the clavicle or back, Spigelia.)

Valvular disease of the heart and aorta.

Neck and Back

Enlarged cervical ganglia. Multiple adenopathy. Hodgkin's disease. Pains in the spinal column, sacrolumbar region and coccyx. Caries of the vertebrae.

Extremities

Growing pains in children.

Rheumatism of the shoulder, affecting the deltoids. Arm cannot be lifted; when hanging straight, arm falls as if paralysed.

Constantly washing the hands; this keynote is specifically Syphilinum, but must not be the deciding factor in the patient's diagnosis. The emotional and mental symptoms and the general modalities are always more important that a keynote.

Swollen, rigid index finger of the right hand.

Oedema of the legs worse at night. Soles of the feet are painful.

Pains in the joints and bones at night, until 4 or 5 a.m.; aggravated by hot applications, ameliorated by pouring cold water over them.

Joint and muscular pains are prone to paralysis; patient cannot sit in a low chair because he loses control over the knees and thighs.

Painful sensations in the limbs of intense cold or burning heat.

Burning excoriation with intense itch between the toes.

In syphilitic rheumatism the patient is a human thermometer, very sensitive to heat and cold, in sycotic rheumatism the patient is a human barometer, extremely sensitive to thunderstorms and humidity.

In syphilis (Syphilinum), pains are piercing or burning, starting slowly and disappearing slowly. Pains start at dusk, peak at around 2 a.m. or 3 a.m. and cease at 8 a.m. with much restlessness and fidgeting. When morning comes, the patient is exhausted and in a state of prostration. Further, the patient urinates and perspires profusely at night, which aggravates rather than ameliorates the condition.

In sycosis (Medorrhinum), pains are constrictive, bruised or with the sensation of dislocation, with cramps, sudden, spasmodic contractions, intense burning of the palms of the hands and the soles of the feet. Pains worsen from sunrise to sunset. Sycotic patients feel well from dusk to midnight. They sleep restlessly (with restless legs) and wake feeling dull, mentally obtuse, heavy and with the feeling that some misfortune has occurred.

Syphilitic patients wake up feeling weak and exhausted.

Sycotic patients wake up with fear and mental dullness.

Skin

Pustular, furuncle-like eruptions in different parts of the body with a liquid, serous pus and copper-coloured scars. Kent does not mention Syphilinum's tendency to develop boils. Allen, Hering and Clarke point out the following curious fact: the copper-coloured, syphilitic scar becomes a brownish-yellow stain and disappears completely if the patient is given Medorrhinum.

The syphilitic patient's skin is covered with reddish-copper stains which turn livid blue with the cold. In syphilitic scarring the skin sticks to the bones.

Finally, perspiration, bromidrosis, the syphilitic skin odour is always putrid and fetid, in contrast to the sycotic patient's odour, which is bitter-sweet, penetrating and sweetish, like the smell of a burned horn or stale fish, a *sui generis* smell which, like the smell of diphtheria, is familiar to every physician who has experienced it at least once.

Chapter 33

Tuberculinum
(1950)

Tuberculinum's main feature is a constant change of symptoms. Symptoms are never fixed but vary incessantly. As soon as Tuberculinum is cured of one ill, another takes its place. Today one organ is affected, tomorrow another. One day the patient feels well, the next day ill. No matter how well chosen the remedy may be, the condition does not improve and the patient develops another set of symptoms which call for another remedy. The word 'changeable' aptly expresses the tubercular state, both physically and mentally. There is continual restlessness with the urge to travel and change his environment.

There is also irritability, oversensitivity and excitability. He is easily angered and bad-tempered, especially in the morning, impossible to please and dissatisfied. He makes a mountain out of a molehill and becomes upset by the slightest obstacles. He will take against certain people and has uncontrollable impulses to 'do something', or break something, to release the tension.

This state of irascibility is indicative of the tubercular state in children who are normally calm and gentle but overnight become angry, irritable and abusive. As in Colocynthis, Ignatia, Lycopodium, Natrum Muriaticum and Lycopodium, any attempt to suppress their aggression brings on trembling, weakness and general apathy.

There is great fear, apprehension and anxiety; fear of death; of animals, especially dogs; of dying if left alone and of committing suicide on impulse.

All these fears are present in patients who are always sad, depressed, melancholy, dejected, discouraged, tearful, weeping without a cause, weeping at the slightest provocation and moaning with unceasing complaints and despair.

There is a great indifference towards everything, with indolence, apathy and restlessness. On the one hand, Tuberculinum patients have an aversion to physical or mental work; everything requires an enormous effort; it is hard work to eat breakfast or any other meal; they have no enthusiasm for anything; they hate speaking or being spoken to because they wish to avoid the effort of answering. On the other hand, they are always restless, wanting to do something, travel, change jobs or occupation or studies; they constantly change doctors; they are full of doubts and cannot decide on the most trivial matters; they are always subject to contrary states; they want to and don't want to; they are incapable of even minor decisions.

Fundamentally, Tuberculinum patients are profoundly depressed and the slightest mental effort is difficult and painful. They must read a phrase several times in order to understand it. The brain feels tired, dull and confused. They magnify things out of proportion or perceive them as strange and illogical, which affects their self-confidence.

In a nutshell, Tuberculinum is characterised by changeability and ambivalent moods, with sadness, melancholy, irritability, anger, apprehension, fear, anxiety, indifference, indolence, restlessness and confusion.

The personality is schizoid, self-centred, introverted and prone to scathing criticism and negativity, thus revealing the corrosive and destructive genius of syphilis, which together with psora forms the constitutional background of tuberculosis.

Tuberculinum tends to catch cold easily. The children suffer from frequent bouts of tonsillitis with fever, enlarged adenoids and catarrh of the fauces. Tuberculinum will do what no other remedy can for these young patients, who generally have tubercular parents and eczematous symptoms.

Paradoxically, there is both a lack of vital heat and a craving for open air. Even though the cold causes chills and an aggravation of the pains, they want open doors and windows and desire to be out in the open air.

There is also extreme sensitivity to changes in weather, and Tuberculinum knows when a thunderstorm is coming, like Medorrhinum, Phosphorus and Psorinum.

There is overwhelming fatigue that is worse in the morning on waking. Patients feel faint, as if they were about to fall at every step. The lower limbs feel very weak, especially from the knees down, which forces them to lean on someone. These are tired, exhausted patients, very depressed physically and mentally and with a poor vital response, an inability to recover from acute disease, especially of the respiratory system, influenza or seasonal colds. In children, for example, Tuberculinum Aviare is very useful for weakness after a bout of measles or influenza.

There is a lack of assimilation, with emaciation, and excessive appetite and bulimia – the patient is underweight or loses weight despite a voracious appetite. There is great fatigue with sudden explosions of anger.

It is not good clinical practice to prescribe on the basis of general impressions but, as with all nosodes, the Tuberculinum symptoms we have described – although lacking any outstanding feature in themselves – constitute what Burnett characterised as the chronic tubercular syndrome. The particular symptoms of the case must correspond to the general basic symptom picture of this constitutional syndrome. Thus, particular symptoms such as migraine headaches are of special significance.

Intense, constant headaches which extend from the right frontal lobe or right superciliary region to the nape of the neck and spinal column. The vertex feels hot and heavy and there is a sensation of an iron band or ring which compresses the head tightly. The head is very congested and there are frequent hot flushes. Headaches appear periodically, usually every one, two or three weeks and alternate with affections of the respiratory or nervous system, or of any organ. Symptoms of mental alienation which alternate with tuberculosis symptoms are an established clinical fact.

These very advanced symptom pictures, which may precede meningitis or the total loss of mental faculties or a rapid pulmonary tuberculosis, are difficult and painful to recover from. One such case was a woman with mutism, negativism and schizophrenia who improved with a dose of Tuberculinum 1M; the remedy opened her mind, enabling her to connect with her surroundings and recover her speech, but at the same time she quickly developed tuberculosis of the lungs, which alarmed her family. Her family was even more alarmed when I told them that the previous mental symptom picture could reappear if we intervened at this point. Anxious to avoid a recurrence of her wretched insanity, her family chose to wait. She was interned in a tuberculosis sanatorium in Córdoba, Argentina, where she passed away. Her organism was not able to overcome tubercular blockage of the vital force in its outward curative path from mind to organs, according to Hering's law of cure.

Another particular symptom is constipation alternating with diarrhoea. Stubborn constipation; sudden diarrhoea. As in Sulphur, diarrhoea causes Tuberculinum to jump out of bed. Chronic diarrhoea is common in pretubercular states. Ever since Burnett's time, it has been well known that tubercular patients are susceptible to intestinal parasites.

Rheumatic affections are also typical. As in Rhus Tox., the pains are worse on starting to move, but once in motion are better.

Tuberculinum is worse by staying still, by cold, humidity, weather changes and thunderstorms, all of which are general modalities.

Finally, the classic particular symptom is the dry, hard and spasmodic cough, followed by a copious thick, yellow expectoration. This cough, however, is not sufficient in itself to prescribe Tuberculinum unless it is part of the general symptom picture of weight loss, tiredness and nervousness, as well as the modalities of suffocation in a hot room and desire for open air with sensitivity to cold and chills.

Other particular symptoms could be mentioned, but none of them are of value unless they are accompanied by the basic mental and general syndrome.

The following is a description of some typical tubercular cases who benefited from Tuberculinum.

A three-year-old boy was brought to my office because of his nervousness and extreme restlessness. He screamed and cried constantly. Nothing satisfied him or entertained him. At night, he would get up and cry or start to sing. He suffered from constant colds, a permanent coryza and recurring styes. Despite the fact that he was always thin, he had a voracious appetite and always felt thirsty. He had foul breath in the morning and was afraid of dogs, crying out in terror whenever he saw one.

A five-year-old boy was brought to see me because he had completely lost his appetite. He was very thin and suffered from various infarcted ganglia, especially the carotid ganglia. He often suffered from diarrhoea and indigestion with no apparent cause, foul breath, insomnia and restless sleep. When asleep, he would grind his teeth. He was always bad-tempered, unsociable, surly and difficult to get along with, and hated being spoken to.

An eight-year-old girl had a fever of 37.5°C nearly every afternoon. She had lost about three kilograms in the last four months and had become irritable and agitated, sad and tearful. She would weep during sleep and have terrifying nightmares. Her family found it difficult to wake her up or calm her down. For twenty days before coming to see me she had suffered from three or four attacks of copious, offensive diarrhoea every morning, the first attack on waking. She had intense pains on the right side of the abdomen while running and sometimes even when walking; pains in the appendicular area, lienteric stools, intense thirst and marked flatulence.

A 16-year-old boy came to see me because he was unable to gain weight. He was thin, tired, exhausted, and could not study because he could not concentrate or retain anything in his mind. His hands, face and trunk perspired profusely. Every morning he felt nausea on rising. He suffered from much nervous oversensitivity and was easily angered by the slightest thing. He was faddy about food, and lived almost exclusively on coffee with milk. For the past three or four years he had developed a dry eczema on the forearm and thighs. He also suffered from periodic, vague headaches.

A 53-year-old man suffered from a very painful fistula of the rectum with periodic suppuration, hot, intense, constrictive headaches in the forehead and nape of the neck, frequent colds with interminable coryzas and bronchitis with copious expectoration. Although cold weather made him suffer and he caught cold easily, he needed the open air and felt better in it. He had an aversion to meat and had become a vegetarian. He was always thirsty, very excitable, sad and dejected. He spoke constantly of unpleasant incidents at work. He disliked the other people there and was looking forward to his retirement. He wanted to fulfil an old wish to travel and live in a different environment.

These cases all reflect some of the aspects of Tuberculinum, although the selection is by no means comprehensive.

Mental Symptoms

Nervous weakness with hypersensitivity and much irritability.

Easily angered patient, bad-tempered, rough, unsociable, surly, dejected, discouraged, mentally and physically tired. Difficult or even impossible to concentrate and understand, must read something several times in order to comprehend; weak memory.

Quickly exhausted both mentally and physically, confusion, tiredness. Everything takes a great effort. Lacks ambition, does not want to do anything; even eating is a chore. Indecisive, full of doubts. Agonises over the slightest trifles, does not stick to anything; wants to be idle.

Episodes of profound depression. Worse before menstruating; despairs of recovery.

Nothing satisfies. Indifferent, hasty, capricious, changeable, first wants one thing, then another, especially during meals.

Complains, laments, whines. Complains of petty trifles. Constantly complains when in bed; cries without a cause, is very sad, cannot compose himself.

Anxious, from nightfall until midnight. Worse in damp weather.

Anxious about the future. Anguish with depression; indifference.

Fear and apprehension. Fear of death, of animals, especially dogs (China, Causticum).

As in Medorrhinum, fear of dying if left alone. As in Mercurius, fear of committing suicide.

Extremely sensitive to all sensual impressions: music, light, noise. Averse to touch; annoyed by the slightest thing.

Cannot tolerate anything white or light reflected on a white surface. Metal fixtures on doors and mirrors in the room must be covered. Cannot tolerate the physician's or nurse's white coat.

Oversensitive to conversation. Tired of life, prefers to die (Medorrhinum).

Does not want to talk or answer questions.

Everything in the room seems strange, confusing; unable to find things.

Surroundings, such as room and furniture, appear big.

Worried about trifles. Wakes with a terrible sensation that something is going to happen.

Much physical and mental restlessness. Wishes to do something.

Constant desire to change occupation or surroundings.

Desire to travel (Calcarea Phosphorica, Sepia, Iodum). Mental restlessness. Wants something different. Constantly changes physicians.

Very irritable, with much nervous tension and restlessness. Wishes to run to relieve tension. Is so tense he feels as if he could fly.

Irritability on waking (Lycopodium).

Fits of rage, nerves, hysteria; petty obstacles cause uncontrollable irritability. Must make an enormous effort to restrain himself from doing something rash. Grabs a chair or the telephone and throws it on the floor.

Fights, throws things or punches his best friend on the jaw.

Breaks things to relieve tension (Anacardium, Belladonna, Ignatia, Nux Vomica).

Uses coarse and abusive language; wants to go out and walk briskly to relieve nervous tension (Sepia).

Feels as if head will burst unless he cries.

Fits of rage followed by trembling, weakness and exhaustion.

Selfish, self-centred, prone to criticise and censor; vindictive.

Cannot bear to have people behind him (thinks someone is behind, Medorrhinum, Sanicula).

At parties, stays in a corner of the room. Stands in street waiting for someone to stop and take her with them.

Sensitive to the suffering of others, to arguments between parents.

Easily startled; easily offended; dwells and broods on offences.

Drowsiness, stupor. Much physical weakness. Lack of vitality.

Sits or stands as if buried in thought but is really not doing anything; in a state of stupor.

State of unconsciousness or stupor with a family history of tuberculosis.

Psychosis or acute or chronic insanity with a family history of tuberculosis, or when the indicated remedy fails.

Anxiety and loquaciousness with fever; intermittent, relapsing fever.

Cursing: Anacardium, Nitricum Acidum, Arsenicum, Lilium Tigrinum, Lycopodium, Nux Vomica, Tuberculinum, Veratrum Album.

Contrary. Obstinate. Headstrong (Foubister). Main characteristic: obstinate, restless; anxious.

Desire to break things: Apis, Stramonium, Tuberculinum.

Destructiveness, scratches when petting or stroking; self-destructive, scratches own scars.

Distracted, mentally weak, constantly changes mood and activity; first does one thing, then another.

Melancholy, depression, sadness.

Obstinate children: temper tantrums, children who throw themselves on the floor at the slightest contradiction.

Very excited, laughing and crying excessively. Convulsions of tears and laughter at the same time.

Intolerant of contradiction.

Excessively merry, sometimes with fits of rage.

Spasmodic, intense weeping. Hiccoughs and sudden jerking of hands and feet.

Weeps bitterly and says he does not want to live.

Sad, melancholy, depressed, unhappy, wants to cry; with fits of irritability.

Discontent. Loathing of life. Premonitions of death, thoughts of death.

Children who talk about death, are anxious about diseases and their health.

Anxiety about his salvation and the future. Apprehension in stomach.

Anxiety in the chest, feels an anguished sensation as if the soul wanted to escape from the body, with painful rush of blood in the chest and suffocation.

Head feels hot, heart feels anxious, which causes him to jump out of bed and leave the house.

Much anxiety of conscience, as if guilty of a crime.

Feels as if an apoplexy attack were upon him.

Bad humour and depression.

Sensitive to music, cannot hear soft music without feeling cardiac oppression.

Indisposed to intellectual activity.

Finds it easier to analyse than summarise.

Mental inertia, cannot cast off previous thoughts.

Chapter 34

Essential Characteristics
(1965)

The following remedies should only be prescribed if certain essential symptoms, outlined below, are present.

Ambra Grisea, with a proven condition of premature senility, physical and mental decay with emotional indifference as perceived in the patient's attitude, rather than through specific symptoms.

Ammonium Carbonicum, with hysteria and a tendency to faint or have sudden mood swings.

Argentum Nitricum, with apprehension and anticipation before a test of any kind.

Arsenicum, with scrupulous hygiene and an immaculate appearance.

Aurum, with destructive tendencies, guilt feelings and suicidal melancholy.

Calcarea, with apprehension and fears.

Kali Carbonicum, with fear of being alone.

Lachesis, with loquacity, jealousy and sociability.

Lycopodium, with cowardice and lack of self-confidence.

Medorrhinum, with hurried actions and a bad memory.

Mercurius, with a busy but dull mind, ideas of killing and committing suicide. Mercurius children are malicious, perverse, malevolent, gossipy, meddlesome, crooked, destructive.

Natrum Muriaticum, with mortification, resentment and desire for sympathy, consolation and pampering as in Phosphorus; but – in contrast to extroverted Phosphorus – Natrum Muriaticum is introverted.

Nitricum Acidum, with bad temper, anger, tendency to violence and irascibility.

Phosphorus, with excitability and boasting.

Platinum, with a disdainful feeling of superiority and pride.

Psorinum, with a feeling of forsakenness, isolation, lack of communication and understanding, despair, anxiety of conscience and despair of recovery and salvation.

Pulsatilla, with compliance, timidity and tearfulness.

Sepia, with discontented feelings about the home and family (in the woman) or about work (in the man).

Silica, with weakness and lack of confidence.

Thuja, with obsessive ideas, hallucinations and guilty conscience.

Tuberculinum, with stubbornness, inflexibility, sensitivity and irritability.

Chapter 35

The Personality of the Remedy
(1947)

Sulphur, Lycopodium and Calcarea Carbonica

To know a patient thoroughly, and to understand the personality of the remedy through the repeated and systematic study of all aspects, is the main goal of homoeopathy.

The personality is the combination of psychological and physical components which express the patient's individuality. This involves not only the patient's character, but also the constitution, temperament, medical history, past emotional trauma, repressed emotions, suppressed physical symptoms, intelligence, behaviour and general modalities.

The homoeopath must take into account all the components of the personality, just as they are represented in the materia medica. Personalities are not the mere sum of subjective and objective symptoms, but represent the combination and integration of all the above components.

A single, specific symptom, whether of character, behaviour, intelligence, temperament or constitution, does not make a diagnosis. It is the combination of mental and physical components that make up the characteristic whole. Furthermore, in homoeopathy the mind is not separate from the body, nor is the psyche separate from the organism, as Wundt would have it. The theory, held by Kraepelin or Virchow, that mental derangements are always caused by physiological changes is not valid in homoeopathy.

The conflict of opinion between physiologists and psychologists is not homoeopathy's problem. Based on rigorous experimentation and information from provings, homoeopathy follows the Law of Similars and makes a diagnosis which takes the whole individual into account. It is the task of future research to understand the way in which homoeopathic remedies act and to discover which are the dynamic aspects of organ response. Meanwhile, psychiatric medicine maintains its dualistic approach, using hormones, vitamins and drugs to regulate physiological functions and psychotherapy to resolve emotional conflicts. Why is this so? Because psychiatric medicine is unable fully to influence the dynamic plane where mental disturbance and cellular dysfunction are the result of disharmony in the vital force. The potentised remedy has a dynamic effect on mental illness and acts as a psychogenic stimulus in psychoanalytic treatment, helping to overcome repressed emotional conflicts and to correct dysfunctions.

Sulphur, Calcarea Carbonica and Lycopodium are three of the main polychrest remedies whose profound remedial action covers a multitude of well-defined symptoms. Intimate knowledge of these three remedies is an essential requirement in the study of the materia medica, not only because they cover most human diseases, but also because they are related to so many other remedies. In the following brief description I will attempt to highlight the salient personality features of each one.

Sulphur is thin, emaciated, exhausted and stoop-shouldered. He slouches when walking and, when standing, looks for something to lean on. Sulphur patients tend to throw themselves heavily into a chair or try to lie down in it as if their heads were too heavy for them. These are apathetic, lazy, careless, negligent and slow-moving people. It is difficult to tell the difference between laziness and lack of strength.

Sulphur abhors sustained, systematic, regular effort and can only work in short, sharp burst of intense but short-lived activity.

The features are delicate, with long, fine eyelashes, shining eyes and lips and red-veined eyelids.

In contrast to Arsenicum's obsessive tidiness and fastidiousness, Sulphur's general appearance is slovenly and dirty with offensive breath and perspiration.

The unhealthy skin flushes at the slightest provocation and easily breaks out in itchy rashes, aggravated by water and bathing.

Sulphur children look like little old people who are gravely anxious about their health. (Mercurius and Tuberculinum children are brilliant and precocious, probably due to syphilitic cerebral stimulation.)

They have lean, flaccid bodies with a yellowish skin and a large abdomen distended by gas. As in Natrum Muriaticum, Iodum, Phosphorus, Silica and the emaciated version of Calcarea Carbonica, Sulphur does not assimilate food properly, is often bulimic and remains thin in spite of a huge appetite.

The more extreme types of Sulphur children are scrofulous, big-bellied, with soft tissues and hypertrophied ganglia. These scrofulous features are shared by Calcarea Carbonica and Lycopodium.

Sulphur has a disproportionately large head, with fontanelles which are slow to close in infancy. Profuse, foul-smelling perspiration of the head and neck which soaks the pillow at night is common.

Mothers of Sulphur children have two main complaints: their irritability, restlessness and disobedience, on the one hand, and their untidiness, carelessness and dirtiness, on the other hand. Sulphur children may be quite unmanageable and resistant to rules of hygiene. Despite their own dirtiness, Sulphur patients have a keen sense of smell and often imagine the intolerable smell of their own faeces.

Lycopodium children also have old-looking faces but do not have Sulphur's reddened nose, eyes and ears, nor the lipstick-red mouth. The skin has a yellowish liverish hue, and frequent dry, flaky skin eruptions around the mouth, nostrils or behind the ears. Argentum Nitricum, Natrum Muriaticum and thin Calcarea Carbonica children also look old before their time.

In summary, Sulphur children have dirty faces, red-rimmed eyes or chronic blepharitis, nasal catarrh, unpleasant body odour and are untidy.

Calcarea Carbonica children are scrofulous, phlegmatic, fat, pale, flabby, large-headed, slow in their movements, slow to walk and slow to cut teeth. The fontanelles are slow to close, growth is irregular and the perspiration is sour and profuse.

Calcarea adults also have the typical pale, thick, round and pasty faces. Parents of Calcarea children will say that their children are lethargic, tend to fall over a lot as if their legs were too weak to support them and that, when they run or are excited, their cheeks become flushed a bright red.

In brief, Calcarea Carbonica is pale, fat and chilly, Sulphur is thin, dirty and ruddy and Lycopodium is thin, nervous and yellowish.

Mental Symptoms

Every remedy has its own character. To understand it correctly is the basic component of a proper diagnosis.

Fear, timidity, lack of self-confidence, feelings of inferiority, aggressive tendencies and putting on a front are mental attitudes that are relatively easy to perceive during the interview and may lead to the correct remedy.

Even though the totality of symptoms is the only basis for prescription, certain mental symptoms are also outstanding characteristics of the remedy. Notable examples are the shyness of Pulsatilla; the stubbornness of Calcarea Carbonica and Baryta Carbonica; the irascibility of Chamomilla and Nux Vomica; the low self-esteem and inferiority complex of Lycopodium; the impudence and rudeness of Anacardium and Nux Vomica; and the childish backwardness of Baryta Carbonica.

The importance of mental symptoms is demonstrated when a child who is naturally placid, cheerful and lively suddenly and inexplicably becomes irritable, bad-tempered, surly, unsociable and depressed. Tuberculinum would be indicated in this case, especially if there were no other symptoms.

It is important to realise that a cure for such mental symptoms in childhood would depend not only on the constitutional remedy, but also on dealing with the family environment as a maintaining cause. Although little is known about the interaction between the mind and the body, positive results have been observed in homoeopathy when the patient's mental and physical symptoms mirror a symptom picture in the materia medica. Homoeopathy offers not a clinical diagnosis, but a therapeutic one. Problems of character and behaviour can be alleviated, although a cure would involve the improvement of the patient's family environment.

Mental symptoms are especially useful in identifying disturbances of the personality. Apart from psychoanalysis, homoeopathy is the only therapy that takes into consideration the connections between disturbance of the mind and body, as identified through the provings.

A knowledge of modern psychology helps the homoeopath to see beyond the ego's defence mechanisms to the true inner personality of the patient.

A 46-year-old man, a lawyer, came to see me complaining of stomach, liver and intestinal disorders. He described the pains and digestive symptoms in vague terms with no clear modalities and with a great deal of unconnected details that did not make up a symptom picture. What caught my attention was the way in which he gave his case.

He would raise his voice and gesticulate excessively, showing a marked fastidiousness and a certain peevish haughtiness, as if he wanted to undermine my authority as a physician. I understood that his defensive attitude was an important component in the case and wanted to see what was behind it. He eventually confessed that he was shy and suffered from feelings of inferiority and fear of failure. He said he had felt intense palpitations with anxiety at the beginning of the interview.

His self-sufficient, bold and arrogant attitude was only a front. He was, in fact, timid, depressed and fearful of responsibility. In order to compensate for his feelings of inadequacy, he put on a proud, domineering front – clearly a Lycopodium case.

239

These contradictory aspects of the personality are present in many remedies as expressions of the inner conflict between instinctive response and social repression. Because the psyche controls both instinctive needs and external behaviour, the many variations of this inner conflict find their expression in mental symptoms. The same dynamic stimulus affects both the emotional and the physical levels. According to Hahnemann, disease is the result of an alteration in the vibratory rhythm of the vital force whose nature, like life itself, is impossible to know other than through its effects. This alteration, in turn, generates conflicts with the environment that lead to depression, compensatory defence mechanisms and physical symptoms which all contribute to the general symptom picture.

According to Freud, the sexual stimulus in its deepest vital meaning (as in Bergson's *élan vital*) conditions the dynamics of the mind and any disturbance in this area can lead to physical pathology.

Both Hahnemann and Freud make definite connections between psychology and physiology in such a way as to present the human being, psyche and soma, as a functional unit ruled by a single dynamic principle.

It cannot be overstated that the problem of disease is a problem of the whole personality. In addition to the diseased organ, the metabolic alteration of the cell, the disturbed physiological dynamics, there are subconscious mental and emotional attitudes and belief structures.

Sulphur is endowed with natural intelligence and powers of reasoning, but his mind is immersed in a dark cloud of self-imposed limitation. It is typical of these patients with their congested faces and rather stilted speech to wish to realise their full potential. Sulphur patients maintain their long-term memory but lose their short-term memory and their memory for names, and find it difficult to understand and associate ideas.

They have a horror of conversation and anything practical, and because of their mental apathy appear to be stupid. The typical Sulphur type – with his delusions of grandeur and tendency for metaphysical speculations, losing himself in religious or philosophical reflections but incapable of applying himself to work – is well known among homoeo-pathic physicians. The pure type may be a true manic personality, with heightened senses, a tendency to hyperactivity and a constant flow of words and ideas that run from one thought to another without settling on a single topic.

This tireless loquacity is almost equal to that of Lachesis, the menopausal patient who talks and associates ideas so rapidly that she does not finish her sentences because her thoughts flow faster than her speech. Sulphur is the excited, imaginative intellectual, the ceaseless talker, with a large ego, sloppily dressed and unkempt, who spends all of his time meditating, speculating and putting the world to rights without actually achieving anything. This is the 'ragged philosopher' who weaves magnificent theoretical speculations, but is utterly incapable of doing anything practical.

Lycopodium has depression with a marked decline in mental faculties, lethargy and dullness. These patients are incapable of focusing their attention, thoughts escape them, they make mistakes when talking or writing, omit words when writing and sometimes even forget the meaning of some words. What is surprising about Lycopodium is that when they are excited or enthusiastic about a subject, their mental faculties can become quite agile and effective.

Nevertheless, such a decline in memory and intellect leads them to feel inferior and sad, melancholy, shy, cowardly, misanthropic and antisocial. They become incapable of carrying on a conversation, for fear of revealing too much about themselves, and they avoid all public appearances for fear of failure.

Lycopodium patients are afraid of people approaching them and afraid of new people, and tolerate contact only with their intimate family circle. The paradoxical keynote symptom is fear of solitude with aversion to company. They need to know that someone is in the house or in the next room, so as not to feel alone.

They are extremely emotional people who cry easily, even on joyful occasions, especially when they are thanked for a favour, receive a gift or meet a friend.

The compensatory defence mechanism is one of pride, intolerance, and an imperious and domineering attitude. Lycopodium patients project on to others the inevitable and self-perpetuating dissatisfaction they feel with themselves – and become angry, rancorous and intolerant of contradiction. In a nutshell, the Lycopodium personality is miserly, misanthropic, bad-tempered, irate and liverish.

Sulphur patients react very differently to stress. They escape to a world of fantasy, theorising and self-aggrandisement – the archetype of the dirty, ragged, daydreaming and grandiloquent philosopher.

Lycopodium and Sulphur exhibit the two basic reactions to stress, the former through rebellion and anger, the latter with fright and flight. Lycopodium angrily rejects the failure he has become; Sulphur retreats into a self-satisfied fantasy world. These are two distinct reactions to the same depressive stimulus. It is precisely the reaction of each of these types to natural or artificial medicinal stimuli which allows the individualisation of each case.

Calcarea Carbonica is the most passive and resigned of the three remedies, although these can be spoiled by attacks of anger to punctuate the pervading mood of melancholic depression, physical lethargy and mental apathy. Devoid of energy and quickly fatigued, Calcarea Carbonica's weak, bland character is incapable of mental exertion and concentration.

Calcarea's peculiar reaction to stress is the fear of losing his intellectual faculties, fear of the night, of disease, the future or that people will believe he is insane.

Calcarea has a tendency to repetitive actions, childish impulses, anxiety about insignificant details, and strange symptoms such as the impulse to run suddenly, which denote a profound deterioration of the nervous system. Nevertheless, the constitutionally pure type of Calcarea Carbonica is usually endowed with keen intelligence and a powerful ability for logical reasoning, positive aptitudes which are unfortunately overshadowed by apathy, inertia and melancholic depression. Because calcium is an essential mineral for albumin and has a stabilising and regulating effect on the hormones and mental equilibrium, Calcarea Carbonica's symptom picture has significant nutritional imbalance and deficiencies.

The remedy is always extremely susceptible to cold, unlike Sulphur, who is aggravated by heat and better by cold, and fears open air because the cold aggravates his symptoms.

Sulphur patients are restless, fidgety and quick in their movements. They feel drained by heat, and stick their hot feet out from under the covers at night. The perspiration is offensive and they feel weak from hunger at 11 a.m. – an important symptom shared by Phosphorus and Natrum Carbonicum.

Calcarea Carbonica is slow and deliberate, very sensitive to the cold and has cold, damp feet, as if wearing wet socks, and a weak stomach.

The hand is bland, fleshy, cold and damp, as if it had no bones, and gives a limp handshake. Silica, Sepia and Phosphorus also have cold hands, but the fleshiness, dampness and blandness of Calcarea are unique.

Lycopodium stands between Sulphur and Calcarea. In spite of being sensitive to cold and full of chills, Lycopodium feels suffocated by warm clothes and closed rooms.

Lycopodium seeks fresh air to relieve his congested head but is better by the heat of the bed and very hot food and drink. He also has the peculiar symptom of one cold foot and one warm foot.

Other remedies also have contradictory modalities which are useful to the physician. Phosphorus, for example, is very sensitive to the cold but also craves and is better by ice-cold drinks. Arsenicum has burning pains which are better by hot compresses. Camphora, a remedy for acute collapse with intense prostration and extreme cold, rejects warm wraps and does not want to be covered. Pulsatilla and Nux Moschata have dry mouths but no thirst.

Most of the main polychrests, including Sulphur, Calcarea Carbonica and Lycopodium, have an affinity for the different stages of life. Calcarea Carbonica corresponds to childhood, when activity of the lymphatic system predominates. This remedy expresses a nutritional imbalance that affects the muscle-building processes. An overactive lymphatic system and problems of oxygenation would explain, in general terms, the fatty deposits in Calcarea's tissues. The child with a full-moon face, and the aggravation of symptoms during the full moon, comes to mind.

Thus we observe fat Calcarea children, who are attractive to look at but suffer from hyperplasia and hydrops, with bow-legs due to deficient ossification, who fall often due to their weak ligaments, with lax tissues, late development of the bones, fontanelles that are slow to close, slow mental development and enlarged tonsils, adenoids and ganglia, all of which are typical symptoms of rickets, scrofula and tuberculosis.

Sulphur is a basic component of the protein molecule and corresponds to adult life, when circulatory activity predominates. Sulphur stimulates blood circulation and brings inflammatory and toxic processes to the surface, producing skin symptoms in accordance with Hering's law of cure.

The release of toxins produces venous congestion and vasodilation, when the maximum possible amount of blood passes through the skin and mucous membranes in the minimum possible time to oxygenate and burn waste products. This brings on the sensation of heat, sudden hot flushes, burning sensations, reddening of the orifices and mental sluggishness brought on by venous stasis and aggravated by standing. It also causes throbbing pains, dizzy spells and raised heartbeat, leading to hypertension, a sensation of an enlarged heart, oppression of the chest and other symptoms. Venous congestion, vasodilation and hypertension are responsible for the state of pathological euphoria, megalomania and metaphysical theorising.

The characteristic fatigue and lethargy, the tendency to slouch and lean on things, and chronic lumbago, all stem from the venous congestion of the medulla.

The chemistry of Sulphur is vast and complex; it affects nearly all bodily functions and produces different symptom pictures according to the period of the patient's life in which it acts. In the first years of infancy it makes a brief appearance as the scrofulous, thin baby, its face lined by wrinkles in what could be called the lymphatic Sulphur syndrome. In adulthood, we see the stimulation of the processes of oxidation.

Lycopodium deals with the accumulation of metabolic toxins, due to inefficient excretion and weakened kidneys and liver. Its specific remedial action lies in the liver and gastrointestinal system. There is liver dysfunction, sluggish digestion, easy satiety, irregular appetite, excess production of hyperchloric acid in the stomach, tympanism and constipation.

Homoeopaths come across numerous Lycopodium cases nowadays because of the large number of patients with liver troubles, especially in big cities where people tend to lead a sedentary lifestyle, take too many stimulants and overindulge in unhealthy food. Thus we have the prototype of the individual who is intelligent, sharp-witted and emotionally overstimulated, with weak muscles, exhaustion, restlessness, emaciation, indigestion and a jaundiced skin. The body and face are prematurely aged, due to the toxic effects of chronic kidney and liver deficiency. The intellect and memory are weak and there is a lack of self-confidence, a fear of failure, apprehension, sadness, shyness, aversion to work, discouragement and bad temper. The compensatory defence mechanism is one of arrogance and dictatorial behaviour.

I have tried to outline the essential symptom pictures of these three major remedies to demonstrate how homoeopathy treats disease as an integral part of the personality of the diseased individual.

It is necessary to remember that although the constitution will determine the organic reactions of a person, many complex psychological factors are also involved. There is in the human being both a desire to be well and a subconscious desire to be ill.

Modern medicine is increasingly able to accept this duality as it learns to recognise the significance of the psycho-organic interaction. Homoeopathy provides a major advance along this path for all those who understand that the purely organic concept of medicine cannot by itself prevail.

Remedy Index

245

General Index

CLASSICAL HOMOEOPATHY

Dr Margery Blackie (ed. Dr Charles Elliott & Dr Frank Johnson), 363pp, 216x138mm, 1986, with repertory, 0906584140

Draws into one volume Dr Blackie's teaching over the whole span of her career, setting before the reader the enthusiasm, learning and deep clinical understanding of one of the foremost homoeopaths of our time.

COMPARATIVE MATERIA MEDICA

Dr Eugenio F. Candegabe, 330pp, 216x138mm, 1997, 0906584361

In this comparative study of thirty-seven remedies, Dr Candegabe displays how the materia medica may be reconstructed through the mental symptoms of the repertory, so as to find the remedy whose action most closely corresponds to the dynamic totality of an individual patient's life.

EVERYDAY HOMOEOPATHY, 2nd Edition

Dr David Gemmell, 225pp, 210x148mm, 1997, 0906584442

A successful handbook for the use of homoeopathy in the everyday context of one's personal and family health care. Covers 116 problems that a lay person is quite likely to encounter and have to cope with, either as first aid or else in a wide variety of complaints and disorders which may not be urgent but where relief and cure are sought.

HOMOEOPATHIC PRESCRIBING

Dr Noel Pratt, 87pp plus 78pp interleaved, 216x120mm, revised edition 1985, 0906584035

Written for all who use homoeopathic remedies. One hundred and fifty-six common complaints and disorders are covered. Clear indications are given wherever it is important that the lay person should also obtain medical advice.

HOMOEOPATHIC TREATMENT OF BEEF AND DAIRY CATTLE

Christopher Day, MRCVS, VetFFHom, 141pp, 216x138mm, 1995, 090658437X

Written for the farmer and smallholder who wishes to use homoeopathy in the treatment of their cattle, both as individual animals and in a group. It is also of relevance to homoeopaths more generally, as it casts valuable light on ways of assessing a condition homoeopathically.

HOMOEOPATHIC TREATMENT OF ECZEMA

Robin Logan, RSHom, 152pp, 216x138mm, 1998, 0906584477

Eczema is one of the most commonly encountered conditions in everyday practice and can pose difficult and perplexing problems for the homoeopath. This book sets out a practical basis for its treatment within the context of classical homoeopathy.

HOMOEOPATHY

Dr Tomás Pablo Paschero, ed. Dr Patricia Haas, 257pp, 216x138mm, 2000, 0906584418

Dr Paschero was a classical homoeopath of the pure Kentian school – he trained with Kent's immediate successor, Dr Grimmer. The book demonstrates a deep level of insight and understanding of the classical method.

HOMOEOPATHY AS ART AND SCIENCE

Dr Elizabeth Wright Hubbard (ed. Dr Maesimund Panos & Della DesRosiers), 344pp, 216x138mm, 1990, 0906584264

This book represents a large part of Dr Hubbard's teaching writing, and conveys her great gift of being able to describe homoeopathy in a way that imprinted itself in the minds of all who studied with her. The final section contains the famous 'Brief study Course in Homoeopathy'

HOMOEOPATHY IN PRACTICE

Dr Douglas Borland (ed. Dr Kathleen Priestman), 208pp, 216x138mm, 1982, 090658406X

The first section deals with homoeopathy in clinical conditions. The second section, 'Studies and Comparisons of Remedies', shows to what extent Dr Borland excelled in leading from one remedy to another, often linking them by their differences or similarities.

HOMOEOPATHY FOR SPORTS, EXERCISE AND DANCE

Emlyn Thomas, RSHom, DPhysED, 337pp, 216x138mm, 2000, 0906584485

Injury and illness are among the most difficult events in the life of athletes, games players and indeed anyone who enjoys physical activity. This book is a reference work for all people who wish to use homoeopathy to help speed recovery.

IN SEARCH OF THE LATER HAHNEMANN
Rima Handley, RSHom, 240pp, 216x138mm, 1997, 0906584353

This is the story of Samuel Hahnemann's practice of homoeopathy in Paris during the last years of his life. It draws on his actual casebooks, and shows him putting into practice the implications of his thinking on chronic disease and experimenting with new remedies. We witness the process of the learning and making of homoeopathy.

INSIGHTS INTO HOMOEOPATHY
Dr Frank Bodman (ed. Dr Anita Davies & Dr Robin Pinsent), 119pp, 216x138mm, 1990, 0906584280

Detailed clinical studies over a wide range of conditions and remedies, including the use of homoeopathy in psychiatry. The author demonstrates that it is possible to subject homoeopathy to the same standards of scrutiny that apply to another branch of medicine.

INTRODUCTION TO HOMOEOPATHIC MEDICINE, 2nd Edition
Dr Hamish Boyd, 285pp, 216x138mm, 1989, 0906584213

A systematic introduction to the principles of homoeopathic medicine. It shows how the homeopath's selection of a remedy is based on a process that is based on the perception of the patient as a whole and individual person.

MATERIA MEDICA OF NEW HOMOEOPATHIC REMEDIES
Dr O.A.Julian, 637pp, 216x138mm, paperback edition 1984, 0906584116

Over a hundred new homoeopathic remedies, for use in conjunction with the classic materia medicas. Some of the remedies are completely new. Others are familiar substances used homoeopathically for the first time.

MENTAL SYMPTOMS IN HOMOEOPATHY
Dr Luis Detinis, 222pp, 216x138mm, 1994, 0906584345

One hundred and ninety-four rubrics relating to rubrics of mental symptoms are studied, drawn primarily from Kent's Repertory, but also from Barthel and Klunker's Synthetic Repertory. Followed by six full case studies.

The Beaconsfield Homoeopathic Library

STUDIES OF HOMOEOPATHIC REMEDIES

Dr Douglas Gibson (ed. Dr Marianne Harling & Dr Brian Kaplan), 538pp, 216x138mm, 1987, 0906584175

These studies differ from any previously published materia medica in their uniquely wide range of insights, combining the panorama of each remedy with a faithful description of the mental and physical symptoms it elicits from a sensitive prover.

TUTORIALS ON HOMOEOPATHY

Dr Donald Foubister, 200pp, 216x138mm, 1989, 0906584256

Offers an insight into Dr Foubister's clinical experience and reflects many of his particular strengths. Detailed clinical pictures, including the use of homoeopathy in paediatrics, with studies on Carcinosin and other remedies.

TYPOLOGY IN HOMOEOPATHY

Dr Leon Vannier, 176pp, 246x189mm, 1992, 0906584302

A study of human types, based on the gods of Antiquity. Discusses the remedies to which the individual types respond best. Fully illustrated.

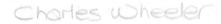